Disability and Culture: Universalism and Diversity

Disability and Culture: Universalism and Diversity

Edited by
T. Bedirhan Üstün, Somnath Chatterji,
Jerome E. Bickenbach, Robert T. Trotter II,
Robin Room, Jürgen Rehm, and Shekhar Saxena*

* World Health Organization, Assessment, Classification and Epidemiology Group, Geneva, Switzerland (Üstün, Chatterji, Rehm, Saxena); Department of Anthropology, Northern Arizona University, Flagstaff, Arizona, USA (Trotter); Department of Philosophy, Queen's University, Kingston, Ontario, Canada (Bickenbach); Centre for Social Research on Alcohol and Drugs, Sveåplan, Stockhom University, S-10691 Stockholm, Sweden (Room).

 Published on behalf of the World
Health Organization by

 Hogrefe & Huber Publishers
Seattle · Toronto · Bern · Göttingen

Library of Congress Cataloging-in-Publication Data

is available via the Library of Congress Marc Database under the
LC Catalog Card Number 00-105123

Canadian Cataloguing in Publication Data

Main entry under title:
Disability and culture : universalism and diversity
Includes bibliographical references.
ISBN 0-88937-239-X

1. Disability evaluation – Cross-cultural studies. 2. Handicapped – Functional assessment – Cross-cultural studies. I. Üstün, T. B.

RB115.D57   2001   362.4'042   C00-931673-6

Hogrefe & Huber Publishers

USA: P.O. Box 2487, Kirkland, WA 98083-2487
                         Phone (425) 820-1500, Fax (425) 823-8324
CANADA: 12 Bruce Park Avenue, Toronto, Ontario M4P 2S3
                         Phone (416) 482-6339
SWITZERLAND: Länggass-Strasse 76, CH-3000 Bern 9
                         Phone (031) 300-4500, Fax (031) 300-4590
GERMANY: Rohnsweg 25, D-37085 Göttingen
                         Phone (0551) 49609-0, Fax (0551) 49609-88

Printed and bound in Germany
ISBN 0-88937-239-X

Contents

Part 1: Theory and Methods

Part 2: Culture-Specific Findings From the CAR Study

Part 3: Cross-Cultural Results

Foreword

The scope of health extends beyond the realm of disease to the wider domain of overall human functioning. Today, the important task of relating health status to economic development demands that functioning and its obverse, disability, be measurable and comparable across national boundaries. However, the move toward international measurement of disability creates significant challenges since concepts of functioning and disability may differ markedly across cultures. For example, different cultures may have different expectations for functioning based on age, gender, and other factors.

The World Health Organization has a mandate to develop health classifications that are generalizable to different nations and cultures, and to make these classification tools available as international public goods. Such tools provide a common language for many users, permitting communication among diverse investigators and policy makers, and international comparisons. This book presents the methodology and results of the first-ever international study designed to provide an evidence base for disability assessment and classification. Given the diversity of cultures, work environments, and health care systems around the world, it comes as no surprise that it has proved difficult to arrive at a common language on a topic as culture-bound as disability. In the development of this assessment and classification of disability, it is quite clear that qualitative research into the similarities and differences of concepts of disability across cultures represented a required step that had to occur prior to the meaningful application of quantitative approaches.

There is inevitably a difference between global and local understandings of health and disability. How can we resolve the apparent tension between respecting cultural and linguistic differences in the meaning of health and providing the scientific basis for an international common language of health? This was the difficult challenge that this collaborative study faced.

The collaborative study presented in this volume not only has provided important data, but also has paved the way for future empirical work. It has developed a package of methods, which are useful in finding evidence for commonalities of human health within the diversity of cultural understandings. It has provided approaches that profoundly impact our ability to look beyond "mortality" into disability as an important dimension of health, and to capture this component into standard health measures. It also has created an international network of centers, which now are familiar with these constructs and research methods that can be applied usefully for future research.

The impact of this research has been felt already in the development of the International Classification of Functioning and Disability (ICIDH-2) and associated assessment tools. These tools have the promise of extending our understanding of health, measuring health, and most importantly measuring the differences that we may make by health interventions.

On behalf of the U.S. National Institute of Mental Health, I should like to thank all those who have worked on this immense endeavour. This book will be immensely valuable to investigators around the world who are engaged in efforts to understand and develop a common language for disability and, thus, to enhance the organization, comprehensiveness, and quality of health for all people.

Steven E. Hyman, M.D.
Director
National Institute of Mental Health
USA

Acknowledgements

The cross-cultural applicability study (CAR) was part of the WHO/NIH Joint Project on Assessment and Classification of Disability (Principal Investigator: T. B. Üstün) at WHO which was supported by National Institutes of Health (NIH, US) Grant UO1MH35883.

It is impossible to acknowledge the work of everyone who has participated during the last five years. No such enterprise could succeed without the advice, support and collaboration of many researchers, centres and participating people and organizations. We can only list some:

National Institute of Mental Health – Dr. Cille Kennedy, Dr. Darriel Regier and Dr. Grayson Norquist; National Institute on Alcohol Abuse and Alcoholism – Dr. Bridget Grant; and National Institute on Drug Abuse – Dr. Jack Blaine, Dr. Robert Battjes and Dr. Bennett Fletcher. They all contributed to the conception and conduct of the study as well as the analysis and interpretation of results.

David Thompson spent many hours in detailed, and invaluable, editorial work which greatly improved the readability of the manuscript.

At WHO, several individuals made substantial contributions to the preparation of the manuscript. Dr. Joanne Epping-Jordan and Rachel Shroot made editorial suggestions; David Bramley provided support for publication; and Rosemary Westermeyer and Grazia Motturi provided secretarial support.

Finally, the research reported here would not have been possible without the collaboration of the 15 collaborating centres around the world where the research was carried out, the data collected and analyzed. Many people at both the CAR and the ICIDH-2 collaborating centres contributed to this effort. Local and international advocacy groups for persons with disabilities participated in the ICIDH-2 testing phases, the data from which contributed to the results reported here. The enormous investment in time, resources and person power from these centres has borne fruit in the pages that follow.

PART 1
THEORY AND METHODS

Chapter 1
Disability and Cultural Variation: The ICIDH-2 Cross-Cultural Applicability Research Study

*T.B. Üstün, S. Chatterji, J.E. Bickenbach, R.T. Trotter II, and S. Saxena**

Background to the ICIDH

Over the last three decades or so there has been a gradual shift in the conceptualization of health and disability. The focus has moved away from diagnosis alone towards an understanding of the consequences of health conditions in terms of disabilities that are experienced at the level of the body, the person and the overall social context. In addition, the subjective components of a health experience ("quality of life," "subjective well-being") have also acquired legitimacy in the understanding of all aspects of health and its consequences. It is therefore no longer sufficient and defensible to look merely at diagnosis to seek to understand the full breadth of the health experience; instead, functioning, disability and the quality of life must also be examined. Moreover, we now appreciate that health experiences, because they occur in a specific context, cannot be divorced from environmental and personal factors that may differ from one geographical location to another.

In recognition of this change, the World Health Organization (WHO) has over the last decade and a half been engaged in a comprehensive exercise of developing instruments for the diagnosis and classification of alcohol, drug and mental (ADM) disorders that can be used cross-culturally and internationally. This work is part of a joint collaborative project between WHO and the United States National Institutes of Health (NIH) – in particular the National Institute of Mental Health (NIMH), the National Institute on Alcohol

---
* WHO, Assessment, Classification and Epidemiology Group, Geneva, Switzerland (Üstün, Chatterji, Saxena); Department of Philosophy, Queen's University, Kingston, Ontario, Canada (Bickenbach); Department of Anthropology, Northern Arizona University, Flagstaff, Arizona, USA (Trotter).

Abuse and Alcoholism (NIAAA), and the National Institute on Drug Abuse (NIDA) – on the assessment and classification of ADM disabilities. In the first phase of this collaboration, the focus was on the development of a revised version of the mental and substance use disorders classification for Chapter V of the 10th revision of the *International Classification of Diseases* (WHO 1992), as well as the development of assessment instruments linked to both the ICD-10 and the *Diagnostic and Statistical Manual of Mental Disorders* (DSM) (American Psychiatric Association 1994).

The second phase of the WHO-NIH joint project was based on the recognition that diagnosis alone does not predict many of the important health care and service planning outcomes that health planners need to know in order to make informed judgements about resource allocation and cost-effectiveness. Diagnosis supplemented by information about the dimensions of functioning and disability, however, can predict health care utilization, needs, outcomes and costs. What is needed, therefore, and what this phase of the joint project will provide, are disability assessment instruments that are cross-culturally applicable and linked to a clear conceptual framework.

WHO has also been involved over the last five years in the revision of a classification of disability and human functioning called the *International Classification of Impairments, Disabilities and Handicaps* (ICIDH), first published in 1980 (WHO 1980). The ICIDH-2 – the full name of which will likely be the *International Classification of Functioning and Disability* – will be presented to the World Health Assembly for approval in 2001.

One of the key concerns in the ICIDH-2 revision process has been systematically to examine issues surrounding the impact of ADM disorders as measured by the extent of disability caused by these conditions. The recent recognition that, if morbidity and disability are taken into account, ADM disorders constitute a major burden on society – far surpassing conditions that kill such as HIV/AIDS and cancer – has catapulted ADM disorders into prominence and reopened the debate on whether there ought to be parity of social response between these conditions and other physical illnesses (Murray & Lopez 1996).

The concept of etiological neutrality, embodied in the current understanding of disability experiences and a guiding principle of the ICIDH-2 revision, emphasizes that in principle there need not be predictable correlations between various health conditions and aspects of disability. This means that persons with physical disease conditions may experience the same or different activity limitations and participation restrictions as those with mental disease conditions, so that it is inaccurate and prejudicial to assume that certain forms of disability are inextricably linked to one disease rather than another. A person may be unable to walk around the block as a consequence of a visual impairment, a spinal injury, a neurosis, or an addiction to drugs.

In addition, disability is now understood to be a complex phenomenon that manifests itself at the body, person or social levels. According to this model, adopted in the revised ICIDH-2, these three dimensions of disability are outcomes of interactions between the health condition and other intrinsic features of the individual and extrinsic features of the social and physical environment. It is therefore always relevant to consider the effect on the disablement process of environmental factors, even when the most appropriate interventions are those aimed directly at person. Thus multiple interventions may be feasible and appropriate. Persons with disabilities may profit from medical and rehabilitative interventions as well as social and political interventions. It is important to appreciate that disability is not an intrinsic or defining feature of a subset of human beings (and as such is not analogous to other human differences such as gender and race), but is a universal condition of humanity itself (Bickenbach, Chatterji, Badley et al. 1999). It is also quite clear that it is inappropriate and scientifically inaccurate to characterize disability in isolation from human functioning, or, for that matter, to characterize disability in inherently negative and depreciatory terms.

It is clearly not enough, however, to create disability classification and assessment tools for one language or for one culture. WHO is committed, not merely to the international dissemination of ICIDH-2 and other epidemiological instruments, but to ensuring their cultural applicability. The uncritical transfer of disability concepts and terminology across diverse languages and cultural settings may produce confusion without a proper understanding of each culture. Therefore, the second phase of the WHO/NIH joint project aimed to develop disability assessment instruments, on the basis of the work being done on the revision of the ICIDH-2, that were applicable in different cultures and could be used to compare international statistics and to better organize health services better. Once again, the motivation for this work, from WHO's standpoint, as health is a universal human concern, scientific tools developed to address health must be applicable transculturally and around the world.

The assessment and measurement of disability has been fraught with several problems. Though people intuitively understand what disability is, the construct has often not been operationally defined and no common standard tools exist. There is considerable confusion in defining the universe of assessment: symptoms and signs, activities of daily living, social support, burden, satisfaction, subjective well-being and quality of life may all be included within the rubric of disability. Theoretical frameworks have spanned activities of daily living (ADL), instrumental activities of daily living (IADL), social and role functioning, and adaptive functioning. Determination of levels of disability has been confounded by contextual factors such as cultural expectations and the availability of assistive devices, personal help, and environmental modifications and adaptations (Üstün & Chatterji 1998).

Although "disability" is a universally used term, in both everyday language and the professional and scientific literature, it is ambiguous. The term might refer to a functional or structural abnormality at the body level (say, a problem with protein metabolism or a missing leg); or a person level problem in acting or behaving (being unable to dress oneself, or to drive a car); or else a societal level problem of being socially disadvantaged because of functional problems at the body or person level (losing a job or being denied a driver's licence). To avoid confusing these three very different notions, the original ICIDH used the terms "impairment," "disability" and "handicap" to distinguish the three dimensions, with the umbrella term "disablement" covering all three.

Early in the revision process, it was decided that the ICIDH-2 should not be a classification of functional problems that people may experience, but rather a universal classification of human functionality itself, both positive and negative. Because of this, and the importance of expressing the classification in neutral and flexible language, the three levels were relabelled Body Function and Structure, Activity, and Participation. Since the term "disablement" proved to be difficult to translate, and "disability" was now freed from its association with person level functional problems, it was decided to return to "disability" as an overall term for all three levels of functional difficulty. The term "disablement" is kept as a stipulative term naming the interactive process by which the levels of disabilities come about.

The original, 1980 version of the ICIDH was the first attempt at an international, universal common language of disability. It was translated into at least 15 languages and referred to in over 1600 scientific articles. Its extensive use brought to the fore the need, in health outcome classification and assessment, to supplement diagnostic categories with aspects of human dysfunctioning and social disadvantage.

Yet, the ICIDH 1980 was criticized on many grounds. Its classifications were said to be too closely aligned with diseases and disease sequelae, and therefore it was too medical in orientation (Chamie 1995). It was also said that the ICIDH implicitly assumed that the relationship between impairments, disabilities and handicaps was causally ordered (Halbertsma 1995). Further, it was argued that although the role of the social environment in the creation of disabilities and handicaps was noted, the model of disability did not explicitly include environmental factors and so this essential component of the process of disablement was neglected (Fougeyrollas 1995).

Much of the criticism of the ICIDH came from researchers who argued that the dimensions of disability, especially handicap, were best conceived as products of the social and built environment, rather than the medical or functional state of the individual. Although the drafters of the ICIDH 1980 were certainly conscious of this fact, many argued that the classification was not clear in recognizing that, because of social prejudice or stereotypical attitudes, or just ignorance, people with impairments and disabilities around the world found themselves disadvantaged in many areas of life and unable to participate fully in normal social roles and positions. Inaccessible buildings or the lack of environmental modifications or accommodations contributed to the handicap that individuals experienced; indeed, many argued it was the social and physical environment that "handicapped" people, not their physical or mental condition. Representatives of this approach, often called "the social model of disability," argued that the ICIDH was not an adequate basis for research into the dimensions of disability (Shakespeare 1993).

In the early 1990s, WHO brought together a worldwide network of collaborating centres, as well as a wide variety of health professionals, policymakers and persons with disabilities and their advocacy organizations, to begin the task of revising the ICIDH. Coordinated with other United Nations agencies, the process has slowly built up a consensus on a useful and empirically grounded model of disability that synthesizes the medical and the social models to produce a robust and flexible construct that can be employed in many sectors and for many different purposes. A preliminary draft of the ICIDH-2 was reviewed in the latter half of 1997, and the comments were then incorporated into a second draft (the "Beta-1 draft") used for field trial purposes. By early 1999 the results of those tests, conducted around the world, were incorporated into another draft, the Beta-2 draft, which was again the basis for another round of field testing.

In brief, the ICIDH-2 presents the following picture of disability. All levels of disability occur with a health condition and within the context defined by environmental factors and personal characteristics (age, sex, level of education, life history and so on). The three dimensions of disability are not conceived as links in a causal chain, but as alternative, but conceptually distinct, perspectives on the disablement process. One perspective is at the level of body or body part, and abnormalities of function or structure are called *impairments*. If, in association with a health condition, a person does not perform a range of activities that others perform, this person level difficulty is called an *activity limitation*. Finally, from the perspective of complete context of a person's life, characterized for the most part by the physical and social environment in which the person lives, disability may be manifested as restrictions in major areas of human life – for example, parenting, employment, education, social interaction and citizenship. In the ICIDH-2, these are termed *participation restrictions*.

The conceptual model in the ICIDH-2 (see Figure 1) offers a complete picture of the functional aspects of the health experience, understood as an outcome of an interaction between features of the person, on the one hand, and social and physical environmental factors on the other. By incorporating both the medical and the social models of disability, the ICIDH-2 provides a flexible classificatory tool that allows users to describe, in an international common language, both medical and rehabilitative phenomena (from the perspective of impairments and activity limitations) as well as consequences of the environment for persons with disabilities with regard to their levels of participation in the full range of human life. Rather than being a classification of persons with disabilities, or even of the problems that they may experience, the ICIDH-2 is a classification of functionality at three levels, understood in neutral terms. In this way, the user can identify, not only problems at the level of body, person and society, but also absence of problems and presence of strengths. The ICIDH-2 is a universal tool for the classification of functioning and disability.

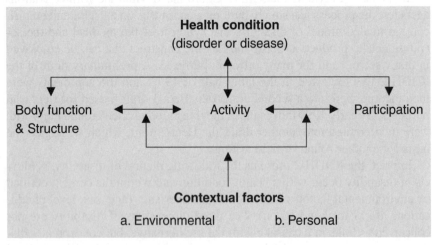

Figure 1. The ICIDH-2 model of disability

The study of disability involves a confluence of medical care, rehabilitation, education, and community action as well as law, politics and social science research. The ICIDH-2 is designed for these uses in preparation for a new era of disability studies. For it is no longer sufficient to rely on one approach to the exclusion of another. Numbers must be joined to narratives. Social theory must have a place along with health sciences in formulation of policy. By addressing the local context of the social experience of a health condition and associated disability we have a better chance of improving the quality of life of people. Health policy is thus inseparable from social policy. Innovations in social policy derived from collective experience are necessary to address the needs of local communities. This is the new world of research that the ICIDH-2 anticipates.

Cultural diversity and universality?

There is, however, a fundamental dilemma that poses an obstacle to this research agenda. It is generally agreed that the appropriate aim of a classification tool such as the ICIDH-2 is to provide an international common language, as well as a universal conceptual framework for disability across languages and cultures. Yet the experience of disability is unique to each individual, not only because the precise manifestation of a disease, disorder or injury is unique, but also because the consequences of these health conditions will be influenced by a complex combination of factors, from personal differences in experience, background and basic emotional, psychological and intellectual make-up to differences in the physical, social and cultural context in which that person lives. This fact, moreover, is fundamental to the background model of the ICIDH-2, which sees the process of disablement as fitting within the complete social and physical environment in which a person lives.

Some suggest, however, that a strong case can be made against the possibility of a universal and transcultural common language for all three dimensions of disability. For not only are personal experiences of disability individual and unique, but perception of and attitudes towards disability are highly relative, since they are subject to cultural interpretations that depend on values, contexts, socio-historical time and place, as well as the perspective and social status of the observer. Disability and its social construction accordingly vary from society to society and from time to time. Throughout human history societies have defined the notion of disability and its dimensions in different ways, and these definitions have themselves evolved over time.

Despite this, as noted, the ICIDH-2 revision process is based on the principle that disability is a universal trait of human beings and not a unique identifier of a social group. The principle of universalism entails that all human beings have, either in fact or potentially, some limitation in functionality at the body, person or social level associated with a health condition. Disability is not, in short, a defining feature of a minority of people; it is a universal human trait. Nor is disability a dichotomous status; instead there is a continuum of levels and degrees of functionality. Disability, in all its dimensions, is always relative to the expectations placed on people's functioning – what they are expected to do and not do. A clear consequence of universalism is that underlying the diversity of manifestations of disability, there must be a core of functional states that are amenable to scientific identification. This underlying commonality is, of course, what ICIDH-2 attempts to classify.

Universalism does not necessarily implies that impairment always and in every society will lead to activity limitations or participation restrictions. To be sure, we have unequivocal evidence from archaeological sites that living with impairment is ubiquitous. Skeletal remains often demonstrate congenital malformations, trauma or arthritic changes. We can assume that these impairments lead to the same or similar kinds of activity limitations wherever they occur. But we also know that it is wrong to assume that impairments or activity limitations cause a person to be automatically marginalized from social groups or to be otherwise disadvantaged by having their participation restricted in some area of life. Though this may be true of a small number of serious impairments and activity limitations such as blindness or paraplegia, these are not representative of the wider domain of disabilities, many of which go unnoticed, or are not socially visible because of coping or accommodation mechanisms.

The variety of roles that people with disabilities occupy is striking. In some communities persons with disabilities are priests, in others they are musicians or artisans. And in yet other societies, they are beggars. When a high percentage of persons with a disability live in a small population, strong cultural traditions often emerge to support the participation of the disabled person in whatever roles the society deems appropriate. People with albinism in the Cuna Indian population in Panama (de Smidt 1948), and the deaf on the island of Martha's Vineyard in the United States (Groce 1985) are examples of small scale societies in which disabled individuals are related and connected to each other through diffuse social roles and contexts.

In short, it may not be possible, anthropologically and in special cases, to generalize from a physical impairment to a single social identity. It might be safe to offer as a hypothesis, however, that in complex societies that stress individualism and achievement, and where social relationships are more impersonal and task-specific, peoples' physical characteristics are more often used to classify people and form their personal identity.

Science, bureaucracy and organized religion have each played an important role in shaping the construction of disability: as the broken, incomplete and imperfect self, as the case requiring management, and as the object of pity and charity. This has led people to argue for a more integrated conception of self, based not upon an empirical, mechanized and bureaucratic world-view, but upon an integrated, interdependent and holistic view of self and society. In that way a more universal understanding of disability may be possible. At the same time, when we turn to the issue of social attitudes toward disability, and people with disabilities, including the way people report disability and its severity, we are confronted with what appears to be an enormous variation across cultures. Consider these recent studies, and the hypotheses they suggest:

- A study of randomly selected villagers in Vellore in southern India, which examined attitudes towards individuals with physical disabilities, revealed that 82% of these attitudes were positive (Bakheit & Shanmugalingam 1997). Gender and employment status did not appear to have an influence on whether the respondent regarded disabled people in a positive or negative way but most older individuals expressed prejudice or challenged the rights of disabled people to equal opportunities in education, employment and social integration. This suggests that in some contexts and social arrangements disability can be positively valued, a fact that should encourage disability advocates around the world.

- In older Chinese society, the support provided by family members, as well as adequate income to meet living expenses, have been found to play a role equal to that of physical factors in contributing to life satisfaction (Ho, Woo & Lau et al. 1995). This supports the view that background social factors influence the subjective experience of disability.

- Doyle and Wong (1996), in a study of Cantonese-speaking adults, showed that they do not perceive a hearing problem even when screening tests identify hearing loss. Among persons who failed a screening test for hearing, more than two-thirds reported that they had no problems in hearing during conversations. Persons who reported hearing difficulties tended to have meant hearing levels in excess of the screening threshold. In a similar study in rural Egypt examining the experience of blindness, it was found that villagers' assessments of their vision differed substantially from ophthalmic measurements of their vision (Lane, Mikhail, Reizian et al. 1993). Individuals with profound visual loss remained independent in their daily activities and contributed to their families' subsistence. While they agreed that they had "weak eyesight," they did not perceive themselves to be disabled. This suggests that the presence of disability is a function of expectations, which are culturally or socially determined.

- A study of the traditional beliefs and practices concerning leprosy of the Limba people of Sierra Leone showed that their traditional definition of illness holds that a person is seriously ill only when he or she has severe pain or disability (Opala & Boillot 1996). As a result, they seek help only at relatively advanced stages of the disease. In a study of low-income Puerto Rican parents whose children were classified as learning-disabled or mildly mentally retarded, it was shown that cultural meanings of disability and normalcy may lead parents to reject the very notion of disability (Ruiz 1995). The parents focused instead on the impact of family identity, language confusion, and detrimental educational practices as causes of their children's school performance. Thus the threshold of what constitutes a disability may be determined by cultural expectations.

- Considerable differences between concepts of disease, disability and well-being between Bengalis and Somalis living in the United Kingdom have been documented (Silveira & Ebrahim 1995). In study on epilepsy in Zimbabwe and the USA, Devlieger, Piachaud and Leung (1994) showed that coping skills in a group of Zimbabweans tended to be related to the experience of "being different," while in the Midwestern US group "not being able to do things" was a major experience. When the study linked coping mechanisms to the cultural environment, two major cultural influences in Zimbabwe stood out as being different from the Midwest: the belief in external control and cause of mental and physical health; and cultural conflict. These studies indicate that subcultural influences may be more determinative of attitudes about disabilities than the larger, national cultural views.

- In several studies using standard functional assessment tools, which purport to measure universal phenomena, substantial cultural divergence has been noted. Studies using the Functional Impairment Measure (FIM) in different parts of the world have shown that, for example, item difficulty patterns in Japan differ slightly from those in the United States because of cultural differences (Tsuji, Sonoda, Domen, et al. 1995). Studies using "standard" instruments used by the Office of Population, Census and Surveys (OPCS) and instruments to measure activities of daily living (ADLs) and instrumental activities of daily living (IADLs) have shown similar variability. In a study in Thailand using the OPCS interview, the disability score of 4.8 (1.9) with a range of 0–10 was found to be unsuitable because of misinterpretation of behavioural and intellectual disability leading to 99% of subjects being scored as disabled (Jitapunkul, Kamolratanakul & Ebrahim 1994). A study in Taiwan questioned whether activities can be calibrated on the same scale as North American activities to make a single cross-cultural ADLS (Fisher, Liu, Velozo, et al. 1992). All of these studies cast doubt on claims of generalizability of functional assessment.

- A study of health practitioners from the Chinese, Italian, German, Greek, Arabic and Anglo communities in Australia used social distance scales to rate the attitudes of people in their communities toward 20 disability groups (Westbrook, Legge & Pennay 1993). Significant differences were found in community attitudes towards people with 19 of these disabilities. Overall the German community expressed greatest acceptance of people with disabilities, followed by the Anglo, Italian, Chinese, Greek and Arabic groups. However the relative degree of stigma attached to the various disabilities by the communities was very similar. In all communities, people with asthma, diabetes, heart disease and arthritis were the most accepted and people with AIDS, mental retardation, psychiatric illness and cerebral palsy, were the least accepted of the disability groups. This suggests that patterns of attitudes may be tracked, and to some extent generalized.

- A study of visual disability among Hamar men in Ethiopia revealed that even mild visual disability is less common in men (Courtright, Klungsoyr & Lewallen, et al. 1993). In Hamar society men have two roles, those of herders or warriors. Warriors with visual loss will be less successful in defending themselves. The study suggested that Hamar men who develop visual loss have increased mortality compared to women with visual loss. Vision loss in women does not appear to have life-threatening consequences. This is sometimes called the phenomenon of "spread" in which social roles extend, or constrain, the level of disability experienced and reported by individuals.

These and other studies appear to argue against the possibility of a universal, transcultural classification of disability, such as the ICIDH-2 purports to be. There seems as well to be support in this from studies in medical anthropology that suggest that many health and illness concepts are variable across cultures and sub-cultures (for example, the studies of Bice & Kalimo 1971, Scheer & Groce 1988, Pezza 1991, Weller et al. 1991, and Yoder & Hornick 1996).

Recently, the denial of the possibility of universality in the case of disability was explicitly made by Benedicte Ingstad and Susan Reynolds Whyte in one of the first collections of anthropological studies explicitly focusing on the social perception of disability. Ingstad and Whyte (1995) claim that, in their view, "attempts to universalize the category 'disabled' ran into conceptual problems of the most fundamental sort." They argue that the supposition that universal definitions and classifications of disability are possible is itself a culturally determined view, associated with North American and European societies with their strong attachment to universalistic biomedical sciences, on the one hand, and individualistic conceptions of personhood on the other.

There does indeed appear to be evidence from anthropology and medical sociology that cultural beliefs affect how health care professionals and people with disabilities interpret health, illness and disability. Cultural beliefs cause people to learn "approved" ways of being ill, influence their attribution of the etiology of illness or disability, and determine what they expect from treatment and their physicians and other health professionals. Consequently, health professionals need to be aware of cultural differences that can affect the outcome of treatment. Yet why should this fact undermine the possibility, let alone the usefulness, of an international classification of disability? Some researchers would reject outright the view that cultural difference on its own can be interpreted as grounds for doubting the existence of underlying, objective and transcultural disability phenomena. These unrepentant positivists would argue that cultural differences are irrelevant, or at least should not stand in the way of producing a universal classification instrument. However, this is too extreme a reaction to the concerns of anthropologists and others.

At least two other reactions are possible. Following Ingstad and Whyte, we might distinguish between "weak" and "radical" relativism. The weak version asserts that the relationship between the dimensions of disability is relative to the context in which the disability is manifested: cultural variation, as well as climatic and physical environmental variation, will contribute to the disabling consequences of similar impairments. This being so, the weak relativist would argue, it is dangerous to generalize associations or linkages between the dimensions of disability. The weak relativist would also argue that, while the basic concepts of disability may be universal, the linguistic expression of these concepts will vary, perhaps dramatically, across cultures and languages. There is no reason to assume, for example, that every language will make the kinds of distinctions between levels of visual acuity that are found in European languages, simply because some levels of low vision are not detectable, or socially remarkable. At the extreme (complete blindness), the phenomenon will undoubtedly be expressible in every language, although whether that is so is remains an empirical question awaiting research.

For the weak relativist, any attempt to create an international and purportedly transcultural classification of disability must be approached with caution, since the temptation will be great to assume far less linguistic and cultural variation than there may be. Being aware of linguistic and cultural difference is an essential requirement of the development of a universal classification system. In principle, a classification that is interlinguistically and interculturally applicable is a possibility, although certainly not something achieved without considerable sensitivity and effort.

It is precisely this possibility, however, that the radical relativist rejects. According to this view, the very existence of disability concepts, not merely their linguistic or cultural applicability, is a social construction, highly relative to culture and historical period. For the radical relativist, no universal conceptualization of disability is justifiable since we cannot presume that any disability concept (let alone the overall conceptualization of disability) applies, or even makes sense, in all cultures around the globe. Different cultures "construct" disability differently (or not at all), and there is no reason to think that these differences are commensurable, intertranslatable, or intelligible between cultures.

The key issue in this debate is not so much who is right, but whether it is possible, empirically, to determine which position is more plausible. On some interpretations, the radical relativist position is non-falsifiable: no evidence is in principle available to confirm or deny the position since it is a moral or political stance disguised as a scientific hypothesis. If, however, the radical position were amenable to empirical evidence, how could we proceed?

The radical relativist may reject this question from the start. Asking for empirical evidence, he or she may insist, is itself a reflection of a particular worldview that need not be shared. Moreover, any empirical method proposed to settle the issue might be thought to prejudge the radical relativist position. If this is the view, however, the debate between the relativist and others must grind to a halt, not because the radical relativist has won a victory, but because nothing more can be said. The price paid for the end of the debate, moreover, is very high. If we cannot move the debate forward, then we cannot begin to address the genuine social issues of unmet health needs, discrimination and other forms of social disadvantage. This version of the radical relativist position leads only to social stagnation and the *status quo*.

There is no reason to abandon hope. On the face of it, it is not implausible to argue that, despite linguistic and cultural differences, a transcultural understanding of disability is possible. First of all, few have argued, or presented evidence, that impairments (abnormalities of bodily structure or function, based on biomedical norms) are radically relative. Most commonly, the radical relativist will claim that it is the manifestation of impairments in the lives of people that is relative. At the same time, though, if it is understood that disabilities are concerned with integrated activities that are expected of a person, and that those expectations will differ between culture, then a classification of all, or an overlapping common set, of integrated activities should be feasible.

But if our hypothesis is that a universal classification and assessment of disability is a possibility, how do we identify commonalties without losing sight of the cultural and linguistic differences and integrate these into the development of these instruments?

The cross-cultural applicability research (CAR) on disability that will be reported in this volume was a response to this challenge. Is it possible to identify and measure those concepts that form the conceptual core of disability phenomena without losing sight of the differences that occur across cultures? What can we learn from the similarities even as we observe the differences?

An overview of cross-cultural applicability research (CAR)

Although the next two chapters will lay out in detail the rationales and methodologies of the CAR research, a few preliminary remarks about this complex, international research might be helpfully made at this point.

As mentioned, the research initiative described here was the second phase of the WHO-NIH joint project, principally aimed at developing disability assessment instruments applicable in different cultures, for comparative statistical purposes. Ultimately, this information will be of help in the organization of health services around the world. In order to achieve this, it was felt that two important issues needed to be addressed:

1. The cultural relativity of the disability construct; and
2. The psychometric requirements for the development of cross-cultural instruments.

To ensure cross-cultural comparisons, it was agreed that a cultural equivalence should be sought for the disability construct, as well as the classifications. This equivalence can be expressed as a function of three specific equivalences and research questions:

- *Functional equivalence:* can one define similar domains of activities in different societies and cultures that serve the same function in different cultures?

- *Conceptual equivalence:* is there an equal understanding of the meaning of disability concepts across cultures?

- *Metric equivalence:* do the measured constructs exhibit essentially the same measurement characteristics in different cultures?

To achieve cultural consistency in the assessment of disability, the process of assessment itself must be similarly understood in different settings. The assessment terms, and their definitions, need to be examined cross-culturally. Moreover, the research should examine the comparable anchor points of disability (levels of distress or noticeable dysfunctionality, which may differ between cultures) and thresholds of disability (when a level of disability that allows a person to take a day off work, or the socially recognized criteria for early retirement or the administrative judgement that someone is unable to work). It was expected that the identification of a common basis for such assessment domains, scales and probing styles would assist the construction of cross-culturally valid instruments.

The CAR study was principally aimed at identifying the cultural consistency of the disability construct found in ICIDH-2, in the context of ADM disorders. To do this, it was necessary to generate and test an item pool of disability terms as well as identify the anchor points or thresholds for the manifestation of disability. The study also sought to identify appropriate assessment domains and facets, and eventually appropriate questions for instrument development, and to begin the task of assessing their applicability, potential use and reliability.

The qualitative methods employed in the CAR study were chosen to provide the investigators with information relevant to the evaluation of the domains of disability that could be the focus of assessment in a suitable instrument. Each domain (as well as sub-domains, and individual facets or items) needed to be evaluated for cultural applicability. Five specific aspects of cultural applicability were identified as salient:

1. General applicability: whether a domain, sub-domain or item corresponded to identical or similar concepts in the local culture;

2. Applicability for translation: whether each domain, sub-domain or item translated without distortion or loss of meaning into the language (or whether a new English term was needed);

3. Applicability for key groups: whether all domains, sub-domains and items were applicable across age, gender, socioeconomic status, occupation, professional group or service agency;

4. Current needs and practices: whether the domains, sub-domains and items fitted the needs and practices of institutions of the culture in order to assess disability; and

5. Social security applications: whether the domains, sub-domains and items were appropriate for local legal and social security agencies and related services.

The CAR study also focused on the general evaluation of the assessment items, that is the clarity of each item and its definition, the utility of each item, and its placement in the classification. The completeness of the item pool was also considered in order to identify missing aspects of disability assessment.

In order to ascertain the applicability of the assessment items across cultures, the CAR study looked into what disability categories and terminologies were in use in the culture in clinical services, social security, primary care services, and rehabilitation and occupational therapy.

In the area of global policy for persons with disabilities, the CAR study sought information on how the local culture affected the process of disablement in the areas of care service utilization and coverage, social security and compensation and, more generally, on the degree and extent of stigmatization of ADM disorders.

The qualitative methods used in the CAR study consisted of,

1. A detailed description of the disablement process in each culture or cultural setting;
2. Linguistic analysis of each assessment item (domain, sub-domain and specific item);
3. Concept mapping for each assessment item;
4. Key informant interviews;
5. Pile sorting of assessment items;
6. Focus groups.

The procedure used for each of the methods is described separately in the next chapter. It must be noted here that though the thrust of the CAR study was qualitative and an attempt was made to build a classification and assessment from the "bottom up," several variations of qualitative techniques allowed for quantitative comparisons. The concept mapping technique, which used several dimensions in the mapping, allowed for the identification of those dimensions that are central across cultures in determining the salience of items. The pile sort methodology provided a quantitative clustering and comparison across different settings and respondent groups. Embedded in the key informant interviews were self-report pre-coded questions that were scored on ordinal scales to detect stigma and discrimination as well as the existence of environmental barriers and facilitators. These approaches proved to be useful complements to the more in-depth qualitative interview methods described later in the monograph.

The sites for the CAR study were chosen to reflect a diversity of culture, language, physical environment and mode of health service provision. Consideration was given to whether a CAR centre had experience in the assessment and classification of ADM disorders and disabilities, as well as familiarity with qualitative and quantitative research methods. Also crucial was a willingness to participate and a readiness to take part in international research and the capability to carry out the basic requirements of the protocol.

The objective of the CAR study was to gather information about a culture's understanding of the disablement process and the societal response to it. It was important, therefore, to identify the best possible informants within each culture. Prototypical representation was sought, rather than probabilistic or random sampling. People were selected as spokespersons for their cultures. Doing so not only provided cross-cultural insights into the social representation of the disablement process, but also gave face validity to the constructs making them more useful in the development of assessment instruments.

In what follows, we hope to show the value of the CAR study in the validation of a true international common language of disability, and the development of assessment tools that are both culturally appropriate and scientifically valid and reliable. We also hope to demonstrate the possibility of resolving the apparent contradiction between ensuring cultural applicability of disability assessment items and the universality of the disability construct and the classifications that follow from it. The focus of the study has been to search for deeper similarities rather than to emphasis differences.

Chapter 2
Objectives and Overall Plan for the ICIDH-2 Cross-Cultural Applicability Research Study

S. Chatterji, T.B. Üstün, and R.T. Trotter II*

Background

The cross-cultural applicability research study (CAR) for ICIDH-2 revision and instrument development was conducted as an early part of a multi-year joint project between the World Health Organization (WHO), the US National Institutes of Health (NIH), and participating centres around the world. The overall aim of the project was to develop disability assessment instruments, based on a revision of the *International Classification of Impairments, Disabilities and Handicaps* (ICIDH 1980) that would be applicable in different cultures. These instruments will subsequently be used in epidemiological research, to determine the nature and extent of disabilities world-wide. They will be used in health services research to discover better ways to provide effective services to disabled persons. They will also be used in prevention and intervention research projects to assess changes in the levels of disability in various communities, where local, regional and national prevention programmes are being tested for effectiveness. The CAR study formed the basis for assuring that the revised ICIDH-2 concepts, and the instruments, could be used to compare international disability statistics correctly and in planning comparable and effective health services around the world.

The WHO team and participating centres have all had extensive experience working with cross-cultural health issues, instrument development, and health classifications. WHO researchers determined that there were two critical requirements for the CAR research. First, it had to provide data on the cultural comparability of the disability construct, the basic theory and philosophy behind the international understanding of disabilities and health proc-

---
* WHO, Assessment, Classification and Epidemiology Group, Geneva, Switzerland (Chatterji, Üstün); Department of Anthropology, Northern Arizona University, Flagstaff, Arizona, USA (Trotter).

esses. Secondly, the CAR data needed to guarantee that the psychometric properties (in particular, statistical stability, usefulness, reliability, and validity) of the instruments were correctly developed in relation to the best standards for cross-cultural and multinational research instruments. These were the minimum conditions necessary to obtain valid cross-cultural comparisons of disabilities.

Cross-cultural applicability also required the creation of classification items and instruments that met the three dimensions of equivalence mentioned in Chapter 1, namely functional, conceptual and metric equivalence. Achieving these equivalences for all elements of the classification and all items of the cross-cultural instruments is the ideal. The principal focus of the CAR research for disabilities was to provide the preliminary groundwork to meet these equivalence requirements; its purpose, therefore, was to explore the consistency of the disability construct in different cultures.

Disability assessment across cultures requires that the disablement process be conceived as a common phenomenon in different cultural settings, languages, and value systems. Investigating these conditions also includes examining the comparable anchor points or thresholds for common manifestations (e.g., the kinds or degrees of disability that make people eligible to take a day off, or the criteria for early retirement or inability to work). Because different societies have different levels of resources available for disability programmes, they often put the thresholds for assistance to disabled people at different levels, and for this reason it was important to determine if the process of assessment, and the goals for using a global measure of disability are comparable or compatible across cultures. The WHO team and the centre experts agreed that the identification of a common basis for such assessment, scales, and probing styles would clearly assist the construction of cross-culturally valid instruments.

An earlier phase of the WHO-NIH joint project (1980–1996) looked at the diagnosis and classification of mental and related disorders. During that project, a set of qualitative methods was tested to assist with cross-cultural applicability research attached to that phase of the project. These methods included linguistic analysis, key informant interviews, focus groups, expert opinion surveys, and reference case studies. The methods helped to explore the consistency of the conceptualization of mental and related disorders across cultures. They explored such issues as how the dependence syndrome was conceived, whether the concept of "narrowing of repertoire" was applicable in different cultures, and how the basic alcohol and drug dependence criteria could be compared across cultures (Room, Janca, Bennett et al. 1996).

The WHO team and centre experts felt that similar lines of research activities would be useful in order to identify the cross-cultural similarities and differences in the concepts underlying the classification and assessment of disabilities. The CAR study was therefore designed to identify the cultural constancy of the disability construct, and to provide information that would assist in developing culturally applicable assessment instruments, such as surveys, check-lists, and screening questionnaires. The CAR model responded to the need to compare how different cultures conceived of, and spoke about, what people cannot do as a consequence of their health conditions. It also met the need to explore disability anchor points or thresholds for common manifestations of problems.

Reviews of classifications, instruments and the scientific literature suggested that there was a significant lack of parity between the acknowledgement and treatment of physical disabilities, compared with disabilities that were the consequence of or were associated with alcohol, drug abuse, and mental health disorders. Therefore, with funding support from the US National Institutes of Health (NIAAA, NIDA, NIMH), one particular aim of the CAR study was to assess the cross-cultural applicability of ADM disorder-related disabilities. This required the addition of cross-cultural applicability methods that would help to generate and test an instrument item pool, check for missing classification categories and additional concepts, and conduct an overall assessment of mental health and physical categories, domains, and thresholds.

The CAR study protocols were designed to accomplish six goals simultaneously:

1. Understand the current needs and practices of institutions in different cultures that are involved in the assessment or care of people with both physical and ADM disabilities or are involved in working with these populations, including the implications for social security and the law;

2. Explore and describe the cross culturally stable and cross culturally divergent views of disabilities, in terms of stigma attached to disabilities, parity between ADM and physical disabilities, cultural values associated with disabilities, and the forms of support and assistance that are available in various cultures;

3. Determine whether the ICIDH-2 disability domains and items are generally applicable and whether identical or similar concepts exist in each local culture;

4. Determine whether each domain and item was culturally appropriate, in terms of the cultural sensitivity of the item;

5. Determine whether these terms can be translated into the local language or need to be modified, either in the original English, or in the local language;

6. Determine whether the domains and items are applicable across age groups, genders, socio-economic statuses, occupations, professional groups, and service agencies.

In addition, each disability item in the classification needed to be assessed in terms of its terminological and definitional clarity, and its usefulness in the classification.

The CAR study also looked at the coverage of the overall universe of disabilities, and the appropriateness of placing the item in the impairment, activity limitation or participation restriction sections of the classification. This required the use of several classification assessment tools within the CAR study. There were a number of assessment needs that focused on the operationalization of the assessment categories required to develop the ICIDH-2 related instruments. These assessment requirements included:

1. The need for cross-culturally applicability of definitions of the terms to ensure that they are consistently applicable, and quantifiable, across cultures and languages;

2. The availability of anchors that would determine severity and identify common points of contact, such as subjective distress and whether the dysfunctioning is noticed by the person, significant others, or society at large;

3. Identifying the presence of thresholds beyond which people are considered to have a disability;

4. Identifying the presence of positive and negative attitudes, as well as available social supports, in different cultures;

5. Identifying the presence, or lack of parity between the different types of disabilities;

6. The need to transform operational criteria into an interview that could then be tested for appropriateness and comparability across settings;

7. The feasibility and applicability of measuring performance cross-culturally, either within actual settings such as work or the household, or else in a laboratory setting.

This is a significant burden to place on a study. However, the prior cross-cultural applicability studies and advances in qualitative research techniques indicated that all of these requirements and goals could be accomplished with a relatively compact set of research methods. Similar methods have been used in cross-cultural research done by WHO in other projects, a number of which are related to mental health, substance abuse and quality of life (Coriel, Augustin, Holt et al. 1992; WHO 1994; WHOQOL Group, 1995;

Room, Janca, Bennett et al. 1996). Thus each of the methods drawn from these examples, together with newly developed methods, provided critical information on one or more of the issues being investigated and at least double coverage of all the goals and requirements. In most cases they provided full triangulation on the issues.

Selection of research methods

It was obvious at the outset that no single research method could provide answers to all the questions that were relevant to the aims of the WHO-NIH joint project. Considerable effort was made to select a battery of methods that would be feasible in the various research centres and would be able to meet the required goals and standards without placing an undue burden on the centres.

The choice of research methods was influenced by other practical considerations. The decisions set some important limits on the CAR study. The timetable for the study was more restricted than is the normal case for qualitative research. If the research findings were to be useful in the parallel processes of drafting and revising the classification and developing assessment instruments related to the classification, then results from the study had to be available in a matter of months. The amount of work that could reasonably be asked of the study teams at each site was also limited. Only very modest resources were available from central funds for each site, so that most of the data collection was performed with national resources available within each investigator's institution or from local sources and in kind contributions. This constrained the number of data collection methods that could be used, and the number of cases that could be interviewed or studied by each method. Therefore the methods that were chosen had to be very robust, permitting small samples and ethnographic sampling procedures rather than probabilistic sampling designs.

The CAR study goals required that the ICIDH-2 concepts and items work in a number of different languages, but at the end of the study they had to be analysed across centres and described in a single language, since English has been the working language for the revision process and the development of assessment instruments. In such a situation, it is much more efficient to use precoded responses wherever possible, rather than demand the very substantial task of translation and summarization required by open-ended, qualitative responses and similar data. In recognition of this practical issue, precoded responses to questions were used whenever possible. This entailed some loss of depth and nuance in the study material, but made it more efficient and provided greater detail for the comparative analyses. At the same time, the centres managed to provide a great deal of in-depth qualitative data and interpretation in their summaries. This significantly supplemented the precoded data and gave a better understanding of local nuances and conditions.

The following types of methods were chosen for the CAR study, based on a number of general theoretical considerations and on the practical considerations described above.

Key informant interview

Ethnographic and other qualitative research traditions have depended heavily on interviews with cultural experts who can describe, evaluate, reflect upon, and summarize key aspects of their own culture. These individuals, called key informants, provide the basic knowledge that is necessary to understand the culture being studied. Thus, qualitative research projects rely on being able to select and interview an ethnographically representative sample of key cultural consultants (Bernard 1995). This type of informant provides information that is not available from individuals who are outsiders to a particular aspect of the cultural core, or who do not have the knowledge and experience to be able to discuss clearly those elements of the culture.

As the term "key informant" implies, the evidentiary status of the information gathered is inherently different in this method from experimental or questionnaire studies where the data are gathered from a "subject." In the informant mode, in principle the data are not a matter of personal attitudes or individual characteristics; instead, the informant is giving a considered opinion on what is true in the culture or in his or her social milieu. The data are thus primarily attributes of a collective, not of an individual respondent.

Use of respondents as informants is also common in quantitative research. When a survey research respondent is asked questions in the form "What do people around here think about _____ (an issue)," or "What proportion of your friends do ____ (a behaviour)?" the answers represent the respondent's best effort to characterize a collective, rather than give a personal opinion. Thus, although it is not often discussed as such, there is a precedent for research in the informant mode in quantitative studies, using precoded responses. In the context of the present study, both open-ended qualitative information and precoded and quantifiable responses were collected from key informants. The criteria for choosing these individuals emphasized that the key informants should have knowledge in depth in a particular area of culture: informants were chosen because they were judged to be knowledgeable about aspects of the cultural conceptualizations and handling of disability concepts.

Focus group interview

Focus group interviews were chosen as part of the study's methodological mixture to provide the individual sites, and the group as a whole with an opportunity to explore collective views about particular cultural conditions. Focus groups are the commonest form of group interview utilized in qualitative research. They are a means of obtaining a considerable quantity of data in a relatively short period, from a larger number of people than would be possible with the same number of individual key informant interviews (Krueger 1994). They have been used in qualitative research for some time to study knowledge, attitudes and beliefs in a variety of social situations. They have advantages over individual interviews in that they allow the researcher to record and analyse people's reactions to ideas and to each other. The hallmark of focus groups is the "explicit use of the group interaction to produce data and insights that would be less accessible without the interaction found in a group" (Morgan 1997). Focus groups are normally lively and create back-and-forth discussion among the participants, based on topics and broad questions supplied by the researcher. They have the disadvantage of providing information primarily on subjects that people are willing to discuss in public, so that some parts of intimate subjects may be avoided or modified from actual beliefs and reported behavioural patterns when they are being discussed in the group.

Focus group interviews tend to produce very good "natural language discourse" that allows the researcher to learn the communication patterns in the community, as well as the key linguistic properties of the area under discussion. This process is very useful in exploring the "language of disabilities" at the broad societal level, while also investigating specific language and conceptual elements of the classification system. It also provided an opportunity for each of the centres to learn a great deal about public attitudes and beliefs about disabilities, in a short space of time, in parallel with the other forms of data collection that were informing the study.

Structured data collection: concept mapping and pile sorting

A number of systematic data collection techniques have been developed in the past few years that have proved extremely useful in qualitative research projects (Trotter 1991; Weller & Romney 1988). These approaches utilize an integrated set of mid-range anthropological theories to describe the cultural models of health and illness that provide a framework for understanding knowledge of and beliefs about health and behaviour. Some of the techniques identify the key social contexts in which beliefs and values are turned into action, while others establish the intervening conditions that either allow for change (protective forces) or prevent change (barriers) in risk behaviours. All of them provide a theoretical framework for determining decision-making and sustainable actions for cultural belief systems, and they identify the key symbolic and communication conditions imposed by cultural systems that relate to health behaviour and behavioural change.

The approaches developed by Kleinman (1980) and by Quinn and Holland (1987), among others, provide an excellent starting point for cross-cultural and within-culture research on health definitions and models of disease processes, and for establishing the basic conditions that humans recognize for identifying, treating, and understanding the consequences of health problems. These are the most qualitative processes, and the methods associated with these research designs include systematically administered semi-structured open-ended (qualitative or ethnographic) interviews analysed through hierarchical coding and pattern recognition of themes and conceptual linkages.

More targeted systematic explorations of mental health and other illness domains can subsequently be pursued through the use of three interlocked cognitive anthropology methods. These are techniques for exploring the content and limit of cultural domains (e.g., free listings, sentence frame completion, contrast sets), techniques for establishing the structural and cognitive relationships of the elements of cultural domains (e.g., pile sorts, dyad and triad tests, Q sorting, matrix profile analysis), and techniques for establishing the cultural consensual framework for these knowledge and belief systems (Weller & Romney 1988; Trotter 1991, 1995). Many of these techniques provide an excellent format for systematic ethnographic rapid assessment. They also provide a methodological basis for bridging between ethnographic and survey or experimental research designs, since they are typically analysed using both qualitative (description of meaning) and quantitative (cluster analysis, multidimensional scaling, correspondence analysis) analytical techniques.

The structured data collection methods used in the CAR study – concept mapping and pile sorting – approach the two methodological questions (who should provide the information that forms the basis for the data analysis? and what are the most appropriate techniques to collect these data?) from a perspective that complements the other methods used in the study. These techniques permitted a thorough cross-cultural exploration of the disability questions tackled in the study, utilizing statistical algorithms for analysis.

Concept mapping is a technique that allows researchers to explore single items within a larger conceptual framework, while also exploring the structure and relationships among the elements of that conceptual domain (Al-

Kunifed & Wandersee 1990; Adamczyk 1994; Domin 1996). It has been shown to be an excellent linkage mechanism between qualitative and quantitative approaches (Raymond 1997; Wiener, Wiley & Huelsman 1994). It has primarily been used in educational evaluation, including medical education (Edmondson 1995), but has also demonstrated power in evaluating medical model transference (Shern, Trochim & La Comb 1995), assessment of clinical programs (Trochim, Cook & Setze 1994; Holmes, Splaine & Teresi 1994), and policy studies (Lord, Desforges & Fein 1994).

Concept mapping is a useful strategy for revealing how people think about concepts since it requires a person to reflect and cognitively map out the territory of a concept, and in particular to think about overlaps and boundaries. If this map can be well understood and compared cross-culturally it can be invaluable in structuring a classification that is close to the way that people think about the territory. This helps to minimize misunderstanding and the misuse of the classification. Also it would help to identify potential areas of confusion so that efforts could be focused on further refining and differentiating those concepts.

The pile sorting technique used in the CAR study is descended from a well-established family of techniques used in psychological studies for testing subjects' clustering of items and concepts (Arabie, Hubert & De Soete 1997; Coxon 1999). For the particular technique used in this study, we sought to minimize the constraints imposed on the informant and to allow the maximum play for cultural and personal variation. As a result, the number of items that could be placed in a sort was not constrained, and a "residual" category was allowed, instead forcing the informant to sort all items into substantively meaningful piles.

The pile sorting technique allows us to see how natural groupings of concepts are made by people. This is important because it indicates the heuristic value of the classification principles in operation within the classification system. In other words, it shows the face validity of the abstract scientific principles used during the formulation of the classification. As an adjunct to concept mapping, it engages people in thinking about the concepts in a manner that can be very valuable in the design of assessment instruments for disability.

Linguistic analysis and translation and back-translation

Many of the theoretical positions utilized in the CAR study depend on explorations of communication and symbolic interaction both for their analysis and for associated research methods. Some of the current mid-range theories from ethnographic linguistics[1] include the theory that grammatical categories are the primary mechanism influencing culturally specific thought patterns (Lucy 1985); the position that meaning is only emergent and negotiated in interaction and cannot be reduced to individual intent or to grammatical categories (Verschueren 1995); the view that meaning is constructed through a metalanguage structure ("mentalese") that is an evolutionary by-product overshadowing the meanings constructed by any particular oral or written language that we might use (Pinker 1994); the proposition that methods for "unpacking" the constituent "footings" or "voices" present in speaker's roles are critical to understanding communication in context, in opposition to the reduction of communication patterns to speaker/sender and receiver/hearer constructions (Trawick 1988); and the theory that speech creates social context and cannot be separated from the notions of "context," "class," and "identity" sufficiently to justify reifying those notions as separate from speech (Goodwin & Duranti 1992).

The ICIDH-2 classification has faced a number of challenges because of the need to translate it into many very different languages, with full correspondence of the items and complete conceptual transfer. It has become a WHO standard to build a translation/back-translation protocol into the development and revision processes of its family of classifications. Examples come from psychiatry and work on the ICD-10 (Sartorius 1976). The need for a common language and agreed upon usage of terms in these classifications is well established (Sartorius, Kaelber, Cooper et al. 1993). In a refinement of the earlier linguistic protocols, the protocol used for ICIDH-2 was designed to produce three types of equivalence between translations: semantic equivalence of denotation and connotation of terms; conceptual equivalence of the position and significance of the salient concepts, in relation to the theoretical model; and technical equivalence in the way each item is used to obtain information, that is, the validity and reliability of the item across linguistic boundaries.

The linguistic analysis of domains and items was intended to examine and understand how each culture thinks about disability. The focus was not so much on the literal translatability of the terms as on an examination of the role played by the concepts in the different cultures and the nuances in the meaning of these terms. This information is the first important step in determining the semantic and conceptual equivalence of terms and is critical for communication between professionals internationally, and for initiating a dialogue within the culture about disability. This process provides valuable insights into designing assessment interviews, survey methods, advocacy strategies and so on.

---

[1] We thank Dr. James Wilce, Department of Anthropology, Northern Arizona University, USA for a review of mid-range theories that are being applied in linguistic medical anthropology.

In addition to these methods, a description of the disability process in the different cultures was also obtained from each of the centres. It was solicited by means of an open-ended questionnaire that provided information on the individual settings in which the study was being carried out (in the form of a thumbnail sketch of the disability scenario in each culture). It provided the backdrop against which to interpret the results of the study and was a starting point to help identify areas for intervention or change.

Specific aims of the methods used

There were 12 specific aims of the CAR study derived from the specific data needed to complete the ICIDH-2 revision process successfully and to develop internationally stable disability assessment instruments. The data were designed not only to describe the local cultural conditions, but also to allow a comparison of these conditions across cultures. The needs were:

1. To create a general description of the place and meaning of disabilities and disability programmes in local cultures;
2. To summarise informants' descriptions of the current programmes, and need for programmes, that serve populations with disabilities;
3. To explore cultural contexts, practices, and values concerning disabilities,
4. To establish information on the thresholds that determine when, in a particular culture, a person is considered disabled;
5. To compare the relative importance of different types of disabling conditions in different cultures;
6. To collect data on the parity or lack of parity between mental health, alcohol and drug problems, and physical health problems;
7. To gather information on stigma attached to various types of disabilities;
8. To explore alternative conceptual models for the classification;
9. To identify linguistic equivalences for conceptual transfer of elements of the classification into local languages, and back to English;
10. To determine whether the proposed structure of the classification has good cross-cultural stability;
11. To provide an item-by-item evaluation of the cross-cultural applicability of each facet of the classification; and
12. To collect data on the boundaries between the three domains of the classification system.

The methods chosen for the study were also designed to help to investigate information on the cultural sensitivity attached to various types of disabilities. The issue of how to ask about disabilities that have an impact on individuals' sexual activities was consistently the most difficult to approach within cultures, followed by other topics that were considered intimate (some family relationships, politics in some cultures, and alcohol-and-drug-related issues in other cultures). The methods were also designed to help to compare the relative importance of different types of disabling conditions in different cultures. Both issues were explored at the general cultural level, through focus groups and key informant interviews that allowed members of the culture to indicate areas of the culture that would be difficult to explore through assessment interviews. They were then explored at the specific item, term or concept level through the pile sorting and concept mapping data collection processes.

Triangulation of aims, methods, and analytical coverage

The cross-cultural methods used in the CAR study were selected to allow empirical testing of how well the elements of the proposed revised classification could address the primary project aims and how well they could provide an analysis that covered all of the different data needs from the perspective of two or more analytical strategies. Table 1 identifies the match between each method chosen and the 12 aims. The selected methods not only cover the needs, but also allow significant triangulation of results, without unnecessary duplication.

Table 1. The ICIDH-2 CAR model: matching methods with data needs

Research Methods (*Types of data collected*)	Research Issues for Project	12 Data Needs by Method
Centre description information (*qualitative*)	Current practices and needs for disability services; policy information on disabilities; values and cultural responses to disabilities; legal status of disability assistance.	(1) General description of the meaning of disability; (2) description of the current programmes; (3) cultural contexts, practices and values concerning disability; (6) parity or lack of parity; (8) exploring alternative models; (9) identifying linguistic equivalences for conceptual transfer.

Translation/back-translation and linguistic analysis protocols (*qualitative*)	Linguistic equivalences for items or sections off the classification; identification of problematic individual items.	(9) Identifying linguistic equivalences for conceptual transfer.
Pilesorting (*qualitative and quantitative*)	Cross-cultural stability of the classification; identification of problematic individual items; discovery of underlying cultural dimensions within the classification.	(10) Investigating proposed structure of the classification; (11) item-by-item evaluation of cross-cultural applicability.
Concept mapping (*quantitative, some qualitative*)	Cultural applicability of items; problems with taboo; age and gender bias; socioeconomic conditions; linguistic problems with items.	(3) Cultural contexts, practices and values concerning disabilities; (10) investigating proposed structure of the classification; (11) item-by-item evaluation of cross-cultural applicability; (12) data on the boundaries of the classification system.
Key informant interviews (*qualitative, ranking*)	Cultural contexts, practices and values relating to disabilities; perceived relative severity of different disabling conditions; comparison between different disabling conditions.	(3) Cultural contexts, practices and values concerning disabilities; (4) thresholds of disabilities; (5) relative importance of different types of disabling conditions in different cultures; (6) parity or lack of parity; (7) stigma attached to various types of disabilities.
Focus Groups (*qualitative*)	Conceptual integrity of ICIDH-2 model, and suggestions for modifications; exploration of current practices and needs; parity between mental, physical and drug and alcohol use-related disabilities.	

Selection of study sites

Once the methods were chosen, it became important to select a set of col-laborating centres that could successfully carry out the study. A careful choice of study sites is extremely important for the success of this type of project. The standard approach requires and greatly benefits from the inclusion of developing as well as developed countries, together with the broadest cul-tural, linguistic, and geographical representation possible. The sites for the CAR study were chosen to provide the maximum comparability and con-trast of language, culture, geography, and institutionalization of disability services.

In the final selection of the sites, the diversity of culture, language, envi-ronment, and health services was considered, as well as whether the centre had previous experience in the assessment and classification of ADM disor-ders and disabilities as well as familiarity with qualitative and quantitative research methods. The selection also took into account whether the centre was willing to participate, ready to take part in international research, and capable of carrying out the basic requirements of the protocol. Many of the centres chosen to participate had been involved in the first phase of the WHO-NIH joint project on the diagnosis and classification of mental disorders, which meant that they also had a history of working together in collabora-tion on this type of project and were experienced in exchanging in-depth cross-cultural information and viewpoints. A number of other sites were freshly recruited for this study and added substantively to the mix of lan-guages, cultures, and viewpoints about disabilities. Almost all of the sites did all, or nearly all of the six protocols, although the option focus group method was only fully accomplished by 6 of the 15 sites.

Another strategy to make the research methods better suited to the aims of the study was to involve the field trial centres during the planning stage of the study. This was achieved by inviting a number of centre investigators to attend planning meetings and conducting informal discussions with them so that each centre saw that the demands of the study were both relevant and feasible. This process also helped to establish a close working relationship between the co-ordinating team and the centre investigators and to ensure continued cooperation during the conduct of the fieldwork.

Sampling issues

The sample selection processes for the CAR study were designed to address a constant problem for multisite cross-cultural research. The research requires a standardized sampling framework that does not place an extreme burden on the various centres. It must also accommodate the need to have comparable cross-cultural samples, and sample sizes that allow both within-site and cross-site analysis of data collected by each method. We used an ethnographic sampling approach, selecting individuals who were especially knowledgeable about their culture, instead of randomly selecting individuals who might not be able to contribute substantively to the study. The sampling procedures used are described in detail in *Selecting Ethnographic Informants* (Johnson 1990). Their selection was based on the success of earlier WHO projects. They are appropriate for combined qualitative and quantitative research designs (Trotter & Schensul 1998; Morgan 1997).

The study design required selecting a broad range of people with excellent and extensive knowledge of disabilities, since the cross-cultural applicability research was focused on well-defined conditions that need exploration in terms of specific beliefs and behaviours. The general approach followed in the CAR utilized targeted purposive sampling (Kaplan, Korf, Sterk 1987). This technique allows the researcher to build strategically a sample of individuals sharing one common characteristic – such as their health condition – within a large universe of individuals who may or may not share this attribute. Goodman (1961) originally formulated the method; van Meter (1990) and Johnson, Boster and Holbert (1989) provided an important assessment of the representativeness of these samples for populations; and finally, Patrick, Pruchno and Rose (1998) compared the costs and effectiveness of purposive sampling compared to four other sampling approaches. Since the CAR study sought to collect information on the culture's understanding of the disablement process and the societal responses to it, selection of informants was crucial for the success of the study. As mentioned, this type of prototypical sampling was designed to differ from classical probabilistic sampling in that the informants selected were expected to be spokespersons for their culture and knowledgeable about disabilities as seen in their culture.

The following groups were required to be included in samples and subsamples for the different methods utilized by the CAR study, at the various sites:

- Persons with disabilities;
- Informal care providers for persons with disabilities (family members);
- Professional care providers for persons with disabilities (doctors, nurses, occupational therapists, social workers);
- Disability experts;
- Policy-makers or opinion leaders in the area of disabilities.

While any individual informant was considered to be potentially familiar with at least one type of disability, the design was set up to ensure that the overall sample at each site was familiar with disabilities associated with physical, mental, and alcohol- and drug-related health conditions. Thus the aggregate information derived from each site would fulfil the objectives of the study, and also allow cross-site comparisons by health condition type. Since many of the sites had been working in this area for a long time, they were able to draw on their network of resources to select appropriate informants. In-depth information on the methodological approaches and the sampling design for the CAR project is provided in the following chapter. The confluence of theory, methods, outstanding research sites, and the basic questions proposed for the study all provided an excellent platform for conducting the study.

Chapter 3
Cross-Cultural Applicability Research (CAR) Methods

*R.T. Trotter II, J. Rehm, S.Chatterji, R. Room, and T.B. Üstün**

Introduction

Revising an international health classification presents a number of challenges that impose a balance between methodological demands and cultural imperatives. The classification must be based on a natural or consensual framework that makes it useful for multiple purposes (e.g., policy development, health communications, epidemiological research, or third party payment systems). It should accommodate significant differences between cultures based on language, belief, physical conditions and values. It needs to be successfully translated into local languages with perfect or near-perfect correspondence of all of its items. It has to contain concepts that are found, or can be explained, in local cultures. It must be useful to local cultures. And it needs to allow correct comparisons of conditions in the local culture with conditions in all other cultures.

These conditions require that the revised *International Classification of Functioning and Disability* (ICIDH-2) and the instruments based on it that are developed to assess disabilities be conceived in a common way across cultures. The classification must be open to what cultures tell us about what does and does not work, while satisfying the need for a universal perspective. This formulation is constantly challenged by demands that a new word be created, and old prejudices not be embedded in the concepts, terms, and language we use to describe disabilities. The natural tensions of the revision process therefore create the need to compromise between universalist tendencies and local cultural relativism, while maintaining each at an appropriate level in the classification.

* Department of Anthropology, Northern Arizona University, Flagstaff, Arizona, USA (Trotter); Centre for Addiction and Mental Health, Addition Research Foundation Division, Toronto, Ontario, Canada (Rehm, Room); WHO, Assessment, Classification and Epidemiology Group, Geneva, Switzerland (Chatterji, Üstün).

The CAR study addressed this multidimensional challenge by pursuing a number of objectives matched to multiple methods that allowed triangulation of data. It recognized the need to gather information on the scope and operation of disability support systems and other social services in different societies, including information on the criteria and processes that are used to assess disability. It allowed us to investigate the social conditions attached to disabilities. For example, there is significant cross-cultural variability in the stigma attached to disability and the acceptability of the participation of persons with disabilities. The study offered an opportunity to measure these differences for a spectrum of conditions, with particular emphasis on issues of parity in social regard and handling of physical disabilities on one hand, and mental disability and those associated with alcohol or drug use on the other.

Since the ICIDH-2 presents a paradigm shift in its definition of disability, compared with the 1980 version of ICIDH, it was felt that there was a need to test the recognizability and acceptability of the new theoretical construction for disabilities in different cultural contexts, as well as exploring the relation between commonly used terminology for disability in different languages and the terms and concepts proposed in that conceptual framework.

The revised ICIDH-2 has been built as a nested hierarchical classification of categories of functioning. Therefore, it was decided that testing its applicability cross-culturally required assessment of the meaning and meaningfulness of the proposed categories, definitions, and logical placement within the classification. This included determining if the different terms used in the classifications were translatable, if they carried the same meaning in different cultures, and the extent to which different cultures shared the clustering of concepts and terms implied by the hierarchical structure of the classification.

The project also needed to investigate the issue of cross-cultural differences or similarities in the thresholds of identification of disabilities. A disability may be a departure from general cultural expectations about a person's condition, behaviour, and social involvement. Therefore it was necessary to explore the threshold at which a disability is identified as significant and considered serious enough to warrant assistance or other social response, since these thresholds may differ between cultures, even when there is no problem in translating or understanding terms and concepts. The following sections provide details on the methods, types, and ranges of data collected in the study.

Centre description on disabilities

Each CAR centre was asked to respond to questions designed to describe the local situation concerning the conceptualization and handling of impairments and disabilities. The purpose of the resulting report was to compare the context of disability conditions across the sites.

The questionnaire used was divided into three sections. Section 1 requested information about the general cultural view of disabilities in the society. It explored the terminology used for general categories of disability. It also explored the presence or absence of parity between physical and mental disabilities in law, public and private benefits, insurance, health services and public opinion. It asked the centre to identify advocacy and charitable organizations that deal with disabilities. Section 2 of the centre description questionnaire asked for information on disability compensation and support systems in the society, focusing on support and benefits available at the specific study site. In Section 3 the questionnaire turned to specific social systems that commonly exist – namely, workers' compensation system, support for current and former military personnel, and general rehabilitation system – as an index of the degree of societal variation in conceptualization of and support for disabilities.

No formal sampling plan was specified for the centre description, though site investigators were encouraged to seek information and assistance concerning the different societal systems from others as needed. In effect, the site investigator responsible for preparing the centre description at each site served as a key informant on the site. A substantive finding from the process was how fragmented local knowledge of disability matters often is. At many sites, filling out the centre description required a lengthy series of phone calls and other enquiries.

Translation-back translation and linguistic analysis protocol

Pilot study

A brief pilot study was conducted for the CAR project at six centres. Four centres were asked to do a complete translation/back-translation protocol for the entire draft revision of the classification. The translation was conducted by professional translators who also had some familiarity with the ICIDH-2. The back-translation was conducted by experienced translators who were not familiar with the ICIDH-2, and who had not seen the English version of the classification before to seeing the local-language version. Each item that was back-translated differently from the original (even when the translator used a very close English synonym) was identified and discussed, and a recommendation for reconciliation was made. This process determined that the majority of the ICIDH-2 concepts and items were stable and did not show significant linguistic or cultural divergence, even between very different language groups.

However, the pilot study did identify two areas where problems consistently occurred: Many problems were discovered in the new introduction to the revised classification, which discussed the changes in the conceptual model of disability for the classification. This text had not gone through an iterative process in its development. Second, there were a number of items in the classification that were consistently problematic across sites and languages. These were domains and items in the classification that were linguistically difficult or culture-bound. This produced two lists of items needing further linguistic exploration. One was a list of concepts and phrases at the conceptual level of the classification; the other was a list of more technical items and their definitions.

Linguistic analysis protocol

The pilot study resulted in the recommendation that the CAR linguistic analysis protocol require each non-English-language site to do a complete translation of the Beta-1 draft of the ICIDH-2, including the introduction. A further requirement was that the introduction, all of the research instruments, and the two lists of key items be subjected to the full translation/back-translation and evaluation protocol that was used in the pilot study. This process ensured the completion of a targeted analysis of the items that had already been identified as problematic (after they had been changed for the Beta 1 draft). It also allowed the centres to identify new problems through the process of translating the complete ICIDH-2, since the revised protocols called for identifying, summarizing, and reporting on all linguistic problems encountered in the translation and translation review process. This revised targeted linguistic exploration did not place the burden of a complete translation/back-translation protocol on the centres, but it allowed a thorough and much more rapid assessment of the classification.

The two lists provided for translation, back-translation, and evaluation contained 44 and 67 items respectively (see Appendix A). The conceptual list, List A, included all of the concept-terms from the introduction shown in the pretest to have posed cross-cultural problems in meaning or linguistic transfer. This included umbrella and organizational terms, such as "disability," "disease," "environment," and "participation." It also included the key terms from the model description and the old classification, such as "activity" and "handicap." The following linguistic data summary sheet provides an example of one of the problematic items, and the data to be recorded on it, from List A.

ITEM 1: Disease

Annotation: Explore connotations related to sickness, illness, malady. Disease is understood as a definite diagnosis with a clear pathology. Differentiated from syndrome and disorder. Illness is more a social experience while sickness is a personal experience.

Questions: Do these distinctions hold true in your language? Are there different words for these different states?

Translation:

Back-Translation:

Synonyms (local language):

Comments/Responses:

Figure 1. Linguistic analysis List A: conceptual terms data summary sheet

The second list of items (List B) included in the full linguistic analysis protocol contained terms at the two-digit level from the three classifications (Impairment, Activity, and Participation) as they appeared in the Beta-1 draft revision of ICIDH-2. The list included terms and phrases such as mobility, transferring oneself, consciousness, and handling dangerous environments which had been shown to be problematic in the translation pilot study. Each of these items was accompanied by a sentence using the term and some of its synonyms. The centres were asked to translate the item, phrase, and synonyms, and provide feedback on any problems. Figure 2 provides an example of the first six items and their accompanying phrases, from the complete list identified in Appendix A.

ID	ITEM	PHRASES
1	Transferring oneself	Everyday I transfer myself from my bed to my wheel-chair.
2	Seeing	I have no trouble seeing the screen in a movie theater.
3	Using special means of communication	People who cannot speak may need to use special means of communication such as sign language.
4	Acquiring and applying knowledge	The school where I completed my secondary education was very practical in that we learned to apply the knowledge we had acquired through various tasks we had to perform.
5	Dressing	I like dressing myself in different styles of clothing.
6	Experience of pain	I consider myself very lucky since I have never been hurt or experienced pain.

Figure 2. Linguistic analysis List B: expert or technical terms

Linguistic analysis report

The linguistic analysis report from each site provided data on the original English, the local language translation, and the back-translation for both lists. The report also summarized the basic cultural applicability questions for each item, and noted any other linguistic problem encountered in the translation process. These data were then compared within and across sites to identify problem items and, in most cases, their solutions.

Pile sort data collection

The pile sort data collection was conducted using 90 cards preprinted at each site. At non-English-language sites, these items were translated from the original English-language data set using standard linguistic protocols. Each card presented one item from the ICIDH-2 classifications, including the item name and a brief definition on the front of the card, and a code number (created by a random table of numbers) on the back, for data recording. The cards were placed in front of the respondent in nine vertical rows of ten cards each. The layout was standardized according to the random number order, to prevention differences between respondents due to differences in the stimulus presentation pattern. The following example is one of the pile sort cards, from the original English data set.

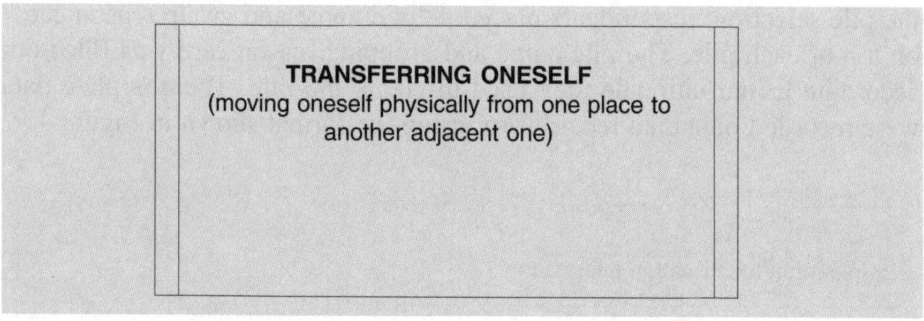

Figure 3. Sample pile sort card

Pile sort items

The 90 items chosen for the pile sorting (and the concept mapping) exercise represent all of the activity and participation items at the two-digit level from each classification. This level is analogous to the detailed subheadings of the chapters of a book. It is the level of detail where it is possible to determine if any important concept is missing from the classification, without overwhelming informants with details. In addition to the activity and participation classifications, some complex impairments from the impairment classification were included, at the recommendation of the centre heads and WHO research team.

Pile sort data collection instructions

The following instructions were given to each respondent, before starting the pile sort:

"Instructions to be read: These cards contain words and phrases that are part of a classification of impairments, activities and social participation conditions. Please look at all of the items, and place them in piles. You can make as many piles as you wish. Items should be placed together according to things that you feel make them alike, and they should be separated according to things that you feel make them different. You can use any reason you wish to create the piles."

When the respondents had finished sorting the items into piles, they were asked to review the piles to determine if any cards should be moved to another pile. They were told that a pile could consist of any number, from a single card to as many cards as they wished. When they were satisfied with the pile selection, respondents placed a "pile name and group reason card" on top of each pile. The pile name and grouping reason card was filled out according to the rationale they used to create the pile. The complete data were recorded on a data record form using the format shown in Figure 4.

Informant Identification Information
Pile 1: 1,3,90, 57, 88, 63   Pile name: [name given to pile]   Reason for pile: [reason for putting cards together]
Pile 2: ...etc.

Figure 4. Pilesort data recording form

A face sheet with demographic information was completed for each individual who provided data for the pile sort exercise.

Each site was requested to collect pile sorts from a total of 30 persons – 15 from among medical or other health professionals, and 15 from among persons with disabilities or caregivers for disabled persons. The health care provider respondents were to include five persons who worked with individuals who had physical impairments, and 10 who worked with individuals who had mental health (including alcoholism and drug abuse) impairments. It was specified that these individuals were to be broadly representative of the viewpoints associated with disabilities in the culture. The consumer and caregiver group was to include both individuals with disabilities and individuals who are the immediate caregivers for such persons. The respondents were to include 10 consumers or caregivers affected by physical impairments, and 10 affected by mental impairments (including alcoholism and drug abuse). Again, it was specified that these individuals should be broadly representative of the viewpoints associated with disabilities in the culture. Sites were informed that if they wanted to do within-site comparisons, these sample sizes needed to be expanded to approximately 20 individuals per group to be compared.

Concept mapping

The concept mapping exercise was designed to be an item-by-item cross-cultural applicability item assessment of the same 90 items investigated in the pile sort methodology.

Items used for concept mapping method

The only change in the items used in the pile sorting exercise, was that they were accompanied by a full operational definition, rather than the brief phrases utilized in the pile sort exercise. Concept mapping has been successfully used in single-culture studies for item evaluation, and that purpose was extended in the CAR study to a multi-culture design. The questions concerning each item and some of the analytical strategies were changed to meet the needs of a cross-cultural applicability study.

The English version of the 90 items was made available to collaborating centres in two versions. One was a paper and pencil version. The other was a computer database, where an informant's responses could be directly entered on the computer. The choice of which version to use was left to the preference of the collaborating centres. Both versions were fully compatible with translation guidelines. However, there were many technical difficulties with the computerized version, which made data collection through that means much more time-consuming than the paper and pencil version. The result was that most of the data were collected by paper and pencil methods.

Concept mapping item questions

Ten questions were asked about each item. These questions were designed to establish the cross-cultural applicability of the item, its correct placement in the classification, and its importance to the classification. The first two questions asked if the item needed clarification in the title or in the definition. The third question asked if the concept could be used without difficulty in the local culture. The fourth to seventh questions asked if the item could be used appropriately and equally for all age groups, for both genders, for all social and economic groups, and for all ethnic or minority cultural groups in the society. The eighth question asked if the item was culturally sensitive (e.g., difficult to talk about, taboo, embarrassing). The ninth question asked where the item was best placed in the classification system (as an impairment, an activity, or participation issue). The final question asked the informants to rank the question, in terms of how important it was to keep the item in the classification system. The first eight questions allowed a yes/no answer, followed by an open-ended question asking for an explanation of any answers that indicated that there was a problem with the item. An example

---

1 *Transferring oneself*

Changing body position in order to get from one location to another, for example from a bed to a chair or moving over in the same bed or chair. It should be noted that disability in transfer activities might arise both for physical and psychological reasons.

1. Does this item need clarification in the title?   1. Yes   2. No
   Optional: If yes, explain or provide recommendation.

2. Does the definition of this item need clarification?   1. Yes   2. No
   Optional: If yes, explain or provide recommendation.

3. Can this concept be used without any difficulty in your culture?   1. Yes   2. No
   *Optional: If it is not useful, please explain the problems in
   using the concept.*

4. Is this concept useful for all age groups in the culture?   1. Yes   2. No
   *Optional: If no, please explain which age groups it doe not work
   for, and why.*

5. Is this concept useful for both genders?   1. Yes   2. No
   Optional: If no, please explain.

6. Is this concept useful for all social and economic groups in the
   culture?   1. Yes   2. No
   *Optional: If no, please explain whom it is not useful for, and
   why it is not useful.*

7. Is this concept useful for all of the ethnic or minority cultural
   groups in the society?   1. Yes   2. No
   Optional: If no, please explain.

8. Is this item culturally sensitive (difficult to talk about, taboo,
   embarrassing, etc.).   1. Yes   2. No
   Optional: If yes, please explain.

9. Is this item best placed in the classification as (circle one)?

   1. An impairment   2. An activity or disability   3. A participation issue

10. How important is it to keep this item in the ICIDH-2 classification? (Circle answer)

             1   2   3   4
        not important   Very important

Figure 5. Paper and pencil data collection format for concept mapping

of the single page data collection format for the first item in the concept mapping is provided in the chart in Figure 5.

The sample specifications for the concept mapping were identical to those for the pile sorting (see above). In fact, sites were encouraged to use the same respondents for both exercises, and in most cases this was done. Where different respondents were used, a demographic face sheet was again filled out for each respondent.

Concept mapping data analysis

These data allowed the researchers to apply several different types of statistical analysis to the items. They allowed the use of factor analysis to determine whether or not all 10 questions were necessary for evaluating the items, allowed cluster analysis to determine classification properties of the items, and allowed simple descriptive statistics to identify problematic items.

Key informant interviews

The research group identified a number of conceptual issues that could be best explored through key informant interviews at each of the sites. The key informant interview consisted of three related data-gathering processes. The first was to ask each key informant a series of open-ended questions. The second was to ask them to fill out a self-administered questionnaire. And the third was to ask the informants to complete a ranking exercise. At the start of the interview, the key informants were asked to describe what they thought was believed to be true in their culture, whether they agreed with it or not, to provide a consensual or normative frame for understanding the concepts being studied. A face sheet with demographic information was also completed for each key informant.

Open-ended key informant questions

The first three open-ended questions were designed to cover the range of terms and concepts that exist in each local culture to describe disabilities and to cover the culture's view on disability:

1. What general word or words would people use to describe a situation where someone is NOT able to do things such as being unable to remember recent events, being unable to speak clearly, having a severe tremor,

or being without one leg, as a consequence of a health condition? That is, people would speak of them as... – what would you say? Any other words?

2. What general word or words would people use to describe a situation where a someone is NOT able to do things such as going shopping, looking after children, playing a game, or showing affection, as a consequence of a health condition? That is, people would speak of them as having... – what would you say? Any other words?

3. What general word or words would people use to describe a situation where someone is NOT able to take part in activities at the workplace, among family members, and in other social groups (e.g., friends or clubs), as a consequence of a health condition? That is, people would speak of them as having a – what would you say? Any other words?

Disability threshold identification scenarios

The second set of questions presented four or five scenarios[1] and asked the key informants to respond to 10 semi-structured questions about each scenario. Each scenario described a health 'problems' that was said to caused difficulties with activities of everyday life. The purpose of the scenarios and questions was to explore the issue of thresholds of awareness of disability, thresholds of intervention, and issues of stigma and assistance for disabilities in the local culture. The five scenarios, to be translated into the local language, were as follows:

Scenario 1 (Mobility). Some people have difficulty walking or getting around unaided as the result of a health condition. Sometimes their difficulty with this is obvious, but sometimes it is not.

Scenario 2 (Mental Disorder). Some people have difficulty with the activities of everyday life because they are bothered by strange thoughts, and sometimes they cannot control their actions. Sometimes their difficulty with this is obvious, but sometimes it is not.

Scenario 3 (Low intelligence). Some people have difficulty with the activities of everyday life because they are bothered by strange thoughts, and sometimes they cannot control their actions. Sometimes their difficulty with this is obvious, but sometimes it is not.

Scenario 4 (Alcohol problem). Some people have difficulty with the activities of everyday life because of their drinking of alcoholic beverages.

---

[1] The fifth scenario is a drug use scenario. This was added at the request of a National Institute on Drug Abuse representative to the Joint Project, after the field research had begun. Some of the sites had already completed their key informant interviews, at that time, and therefore there is no drug scenario data for those sites.

They seem unable to control how much they drink. Sometimes the difficulty with this is obvious, but sometimes it is not.

Scenario 5 (Heroin problem). Some people have difficulty with the activities of everyday life because of their taking drugs. They seem unable to control the amount of drugs they take and how often they take the drugs. Sometimes the difficulty with this is obvious, but sometimes it is not.

Each scenario was presented to the key informant, and a set of questions was asked about the scenario. Then the second scenario was presented, and the same set of questions asked, until all scenarios had been investigated. The questions asked about each scenario were these:

a. If someone had a problem like this, but it was quite mild, what aspects of the person's behavior might *first* attract the attention or notice of others, such as family members, neighbors or co-workers?

b. What if the problem was fairly serious – what would people consider to be signs of that (i.e., a serious problem)?

c. What would people consider to be signs that this person needed help from someone else with the activities of everyday life?

d. How much do you think a fairly serious problem of this sort would affect the person's ability to get a job or do productive work?

e. What about the ability to get married and have a family – how much would that be affected if the person had a fairly serious poblem like this?

f. Suppose a person with a serious problem like this felt that they should get social assistance from the government because of it. What would people feel should be the *minimum period* for which the problem should have existed before they can receive assistance?

g. Would people around here think they should get this assistance if the problem was serious?

Yes   No   It depends – on what? (please specify below)

h. What types of problems do you think a person with a serious problem like this might experience in their daily activities? Any other problems?

[Scenarios 1 & 2 only] What about if their problem was something they had had from birth – would that affect how others thought of the problem and how the person was regarded? In what ways?

[Scenarios 4 & 5 only] What about if the problem was seen as the being the result of a death in the family – would that affect how others thought of the problem and how the person was regarded? In what ways?

[Scenarios 1 & 2 only] What about if the problem resulted from a road accident – would that affect how others thought of the problem and how the person was regarded? In what ways?

The centre principal investigators were asked to provide a qualitative summary in English of responses to these scenarios and to the first three questions (above), in a question-by-question summary of the responses from all the informants. The summaries were to include the full range of responses, and the most normative responses. Quotations that exemplified the most salient issues were requested for each question summary.

Ranking exercise method

After the first portion of the key informant interview was completed, each informant was asked to take 17 cards, each with a different health condition and description of that condition, and rank them from the most disabling (1) to the least disabling (17). Each person was asked to think of the most disabling condition as the one where the person with that condition would find carrying on the activities of daily life (such as eating a meal or getting around) difficult, and the least disabling would be that which would not interfere with these activities.

The 17 health conditions and descriptions were presented as follows:

Active psychosis:	Being unable to judge what is real such as having delusions (false firm beliefs), hearing voices, and being unable to speak in clear sentences;
Alcoholism:	Drinking excessively and being unable to control one's drinking, even though it causes problem in one's life;
Below-the-knee amputation:	One leg is amputated below the knee; assuming no artificial leg, but having crutches;
Dementia:	Multiple cognitive deficits that include problems with memory mainly and in addition with language and with performing motor tasks in spite of no weakness or abnormalities of sensation;
Drug dependence:	Taking drugs excessively and being unable to control one's drug-taking, even though it causes problems in one's life;
HIV positive:	Being infected with the virus that causes AIDS, and may be fatal;
Incontinence:	Leaking of urine and/or faeces with the associated odour;
Infertility:	Being unable to have a child; assuming it is desired;

Major depression:	The loss of interest or pleasure in nearly all activities; decreased energy; feelings of worthlessness; difficulty in thinking, concentrating, and making decisions;
Mild mental Retardation:	An adult having a mental age range between 9 and 12 years; having lower than normal intelligence (say between 55%–70% of average adult intelligence);
Paraplegia:	The lower half of the body is paralysed, including both legs; assuming access to a basic wheelchair or similar device to assist mobility;
Quadriplegia:	Both legs and both arms are paralysed; assuming access to a basic wheelchair or similar device to assist mobility;
Rheumatoid arthritis:	Stiffness of small joints of the hand, more so during the early part of the day, associated with deformities;
Severe migraines:	Having continuous severe headaches for one year and often being bed-ridden as a result;
Total blindness:	Being unable to see at all;
Total deafness:	Being unable to hear at all;
Vitiligo on face:	Having at least 10% of the face afflicted with permanent depigmentation (white patches).

The rankings were collected on a data form for each of the Key Informants, along with a demographic face sheet and the open-ended question data.

Scenarios on cultural barriers and acceptance

Key informants were then asked to fill out a self-administered questionnaire. The questionnaire consisted of two sections. In section 1, the key informant was presented with five scenarios, parallel to the ones in the semi-structured interview:

Scenario 1. Think of a person who is confined to a wheelchair because of a spinal cord injury. The person gets around in the wheelchair, but an attendant has to take care of most everyday tasks, such as personal grooming.

Scenario 2. Think of a person who was born with low intelligence. The person has a very sweet disposition, and can wash and go to the toilet without help, talk to and understand others, and get around alone. However, the person cannot count the amount of change from buying something, and has never learned to read well.

Scenario 3. Now think of a person who says there are voices talking to him/her all the time. Sometimes the person goes up to strangers on the street and shouts things at them that do not make much sense.

Scenario 4. What about a person who can be found in the neighbourhood bar at just about any time of day or night, with a drink in hand. Sometimes the bartender has to wake the person when the bar closes.

Scenario 5. What about a person who can be found in the neighbourhood just about any time of day or night, quite clearly under the influence of drugs. Sometimes someone finds the person by the roadside and has to help the person home.

For each scenario, the informants were asked to check off precoded answers to two questions for each of 10 activities. For the first question, "How surprised would people be if this person did this activity?" the response categories ranged from "not at all surprised" to "a little surprised," "surprised," and "very surprised." For the second question, "Is it likely that anyone would place restrictions or barriers on the person doing this?" the response categories were "very unlikely (that there would be restrictions or barriers)," "somewhat unlikely," "somewhat likely," and "very likely." The 10 activities that were explored were all activities from ICIDH-2, as follows:

1. Keeping things tidy in the home;

2. Using public transportation;

3. Being in love;

4. Having sex as part of a relationship with someone;

5. Actively taking on parenting roles;

6. Actively taking part in community fairs and festivals;

7. Managing their own money;

8. Getting an apartment or somewhere to live;

9. Keeping a full-time job;

10. Being elected or named to a position in local government.

Social disapproval and reaction to public appearance

Finally, in section 2 of the self-administered questionnaire informants were asked to fill out two matrices of questions. In the first, they were asked to indicate the degree of social disapproval and negative reaction – scored by 0 for no disapproval and 10 for an extreme level of disapproval – experienced by a person labelled as being, or having the condition of

Wheel chair bound

Borderline intelligence

Alcoholism
Drug addiction
HIV positive
Dementia
Homeless
Criminal record for burglary
Depression
Blindness
Leprosy
Chronic mental disorder
Dirty and unkempt
Inability to read
Obese
Someone who does not take care of their children
Facial disfigurement
Someone who cannot hold down a job

Finally, in the second matrix, informants were asked to indicate "how people in [your] society would think about the person with the condition appearing in public – for instance, in a store or market." Response choices for the 10 listed conditions were as follows:

- People would think there was no issue, and would pay no attention;
- People would notice, but would not think there was any issue;
- People would be uneasy about it, but would probably not do anything;
- People would be uneasy about it, and try to avoid the person;
- People would think it was wrong, and might say something about it;
- People would think it was wrong, and would try to stop it.

The conditions asked about were as follows:
- Someone with a chronic mental disorder who "acts out";
- A woman in her 8th month of pregnancy;
- A person in a wheelchair;
- A person who is intellectually "slow";
- Someone who is dirty and unkempt;
- Someone with a face disfigured from burns;
- An obese person;
- Someone who is visibly is under the influence of drugs;
- Someone who is blind.

Key informant sampling issues

The research collaborators decided that the set of individuals interviewed for the key informant study should be different from the set interviewed in the pile sort and concept mapping study. A total of 15 individuals were to be chosen for the key informant interviews, divided into five subsamples. The individuals chosen for each subsample were to be as broadly representative of all of the viewpoints about disabilities as possible. The sample was to include three individuals who were medical professionals, three disability specialists, three with a disabling condition, three care-givers to persons with disabilities, and three policy makers or opinion leaders in the field of disability services.

Focus groups

Each site was asked to conduct two out of three possible focus group studies. The first study option explored the underlying model of the ICIDH-2. The focus groups were conducted with health and social service professionals who would be involved in the use and dissemination of the ICIDH-2, and with persons with disabilities. The second study option explored the stigma attached to disabilities in each culture. These focus groups were conducted with groups of persons with disabilities, and with groups of family members of persons with disabilities. The third study option explored the current practices and needs related to disabilities. These focus groups were conducted with individuals who had experienced disabilities, members of families with such individuals, and health and social service professionals in disability service systems. The study explored the configuration of services that were available, those that were not available but perceived to be needed, and the conditions that had an impact on both the services and the need for services in the society. The focus group guides (questions and probes used at all sites) are available from WHO in Geneva. The basic issues covered in each of the focus groups are summarized below.

Focus group studies

The focus group studies agreed upon by the research centres are as follows:

Study 1: The model of the disablement process in the ICIDH-2. The purpose of this effort was to provide a cross-cultural assessment of the concepts and relationships used to create the structure of the ICIDH-2. The primary subject areas covered in the focus groups were: (1) an evaluation of the disablement process model proposed in the ICIDH-2 Beta 1; and (2) an exploration of the system used in the local culture to determine the presence and severity of disabilities. The discussion of disability thresholds, including discussions of the difference between classification of the presence or absence of disabilities, compared with systems that assign levels of disabilities (percentage disabled) formed a part of these focus groups.

Study 2: Parity and stigmatization of disabilities. This study permitted a cross-cultural comparison of the ways in which individuals with disabilities are viewed, assisted, potentially stigmatized, and allowed or denied access to social participation within various cultures. Parity in the provision of health and other resources means that services and benefits are provided on the basis of need, rather than on whether the underlying health condition is physical, mental or an alcohol or drug abuse disorder. The aim of this study was to gather information about the degree to which parity is viewed as a good or desirable thing for society to achieve. The project was targeted at gaining information from college students as surrogates for the educated general public in each culture, and from family members of individuals who had disabilities. This provided the opportunity to add the viewpoint of family members and of the general population as a supplementary part of the overall cross-cultural assessment of disabilities. The sampling strategy also allowed general popular views to be contrasted with the views of family members of individuals with disabilities.

Study 3: Current practices and needs. The purpose of this study was to explore the range and variation in the services provided to persons with disabilities, and to identify similarities and differences in the perceived need for additional services, across cultures. The primary subject areas to be explored in each culture were: (1) a discussion of the existing laws and social programmes that provide assistance for individuals with disabilities; (2) the met and unmet needs for disability services, from the individual and family level to the societal level; and (3) current practices and needs associated with disabilities.

Sample size and resource commitment

The requested effort for the focus group project was to conduct a minimum of two focus groups for each of two studies. Each focus group was to consist of 6-8 persons. Each focus group study had slightly different requirements for the selection of participants, but in each case – as explained above – the participation was to include individuals who were experienced in disabilities (including persons with disabilities, care-givers, and where appropriate, health professionals). A face sheet with demographic information was completed for each person participating in a focus group.

CAR study samples from centres

Each of the collaborating centres completed the core tasks for the CAR study, although some methods were not conducted at certain centres. Table 1 sets out the final data set summaries by research method, showing the overall number of centres, informants, respondents, or group sessions involved in each.

Table 1. Data-collection methods and numbers of centres, informants or data collection sessions

Method	Total number (all centres)
Centre descriptive	15 centres[2]
Translation and linguistic analysis	12 centres (3 used original English version)
Pile sorting	450 informants at 19 centres
Concept mapping	441 informants at 18 centres
Key informant interviews	230 informants at 18 centres
Focus groups	22 focus groups at 7 centres

Discussion

The CAR suite of methods combines the collection of qualitative and quantitative data. Each method was targeted at resolving multiple questions or issues confronting the ICIDH-2 revision process and the development of cross-culturally applicable assessment instruments. The overall results, described in detail in later chapters, was very useful in the revision of the ICIDH, and valuable in the construction of ICIDH-2 related assessment instruments. The amount of data that was produced was enormous. The initial use of the data to inform the revision of the ICIDH-2 is also described below. The data from each research methods at each centre are presented separately in subsequent chapters. Anecdotal reports from each of the participating centres indicate that several of the methods produced unexpected learning opportunities, beyond the simple data collection. The pile sorting exercise was thought

---

[2] The centre report for Tunisia and Egypt were provided as a single report.

to be fun by many participants. It also provided interesting additional information about the classification, because of people's natural tendency to talk to themselves or to the interviewer while doing the pile sorting. The focus groups were particularly powerful in providing the centre researchers with insights into the public's and professionals' views of disabilities in their culture; people tend to engage in interactive dialogues in focus group situations and this provides emotive information, in addition to information about cultural values and beliefs.

By means of triangulation from different methodologies, the data sets provided a good convergent confirmation of many of the findings. In combination, the linguistic analysis, pile sorting data and the concept mapping data identified the items in the classification that are the most stable across cultures, and those items that are the most problematic. These findings have been taken into account in the subsequent development of instruments. The triangulation also identified the boundary areas between the three dimensions of the classification, and the items that needed improvement in order to move from a stable to a highly stable status within the system.

In summary, this combination of ethnographic, rapid assessment, and statistical methods has produced the results needed at each stage of the ICIDH revision process. The methods promise to continue to provide valuable recommendations, interpretations, and innovative directions throughout the revision process to the final adoption of the revised ICIDH-2 by the World Health Assembly.

Appendix A. Linguistic analysis protocol

List A

Disease
Disorder
Health Condition
Impairment
Disability
Disablement
Handicap
Participation
Environment
Context
Consequence
Ability
Activity
Integrity

Structure
Function
Interference
Well-being
Quality of life
Community
Society
Mobility
Memory
Attention
Thought, abstraction, judgement, and related executive functions
Leisure and leisure activities
Economic self-sufficiency
Non-verbal communication
Perception
Civic and community life
Tolerance in relationship
Organizing daily routine
Temperament and personality
Orientation
Self-care
Consciousness
Expressing empathy
Problem solving
Use of humor
Affect
Interpersonal and social relationship
Managing close personal relationships
Handling everyday physical environment
Citizenship responsibilities

List B

ID	Item	Phrases
1	Transferring oneself	Everyday I transfer myself from my bed to my wheelchair.
2	Seeing	I have no trouble seeing the screen in a movie theatre.
3	Using special means of communication	People who cannot speak may need to use special means of communication such as sign language.
4	Acquiring and applying knowledge	The school where I completed my secondary education was very practical in that we learned to apply the knowledge we had acquired through various tasks we had to perform.
5	Dressing	I like dressing myself in different styles of clothing.
6	Experience of pain	I consider myself very lucky since I have never been hurt or experienced any pain.

7	Interacting with an equal/ co-worker/peer	The atmosphere at my place of work is wonderful, the interactions between peers and co-workers are cooperative, generally fruitful and pleasant.
8	Recognizing directions in space and time	I have no difficulty recognizing directions in space and time, I always know where I am going even in foreign cities and I have a very good notion of the sequence and occurrence of events.
9	Keeping appropriate physical contact, and maintenance of social space	I wish other people would keep to appropriate physical contact, I don't being touched by others even if they are just trying to be friendly. I also don't like people getting too close to me, I like to maintain my social space.
10	Understanding specific signs	I have no problem understanding specific signs when looking for the toilet in a restaurant or other public place.
11	Visual sensory functions	I use my visual sensory functions to see things that are near and far clearly.
12	Use of communication devices	I feel very uncomfortable using communication devices like the telephone.
13	Keeping self clean and appropriately groomed	It is pleasant to begin the day having washed, feeling fresh, and keeping oneself clean and appropriately groomed.
14	Hearing	I have no difficulty hearing somebody call my name from the next room.
15	Hearing functions	My hearing functions are not good enough to be able to hear soft sounds or whispers.
16	Taking care of one's health	I take care of my health by having regular medical check ups and following what my doctor tells me to do.
17	Eating and drinking	I like eating and drinking tasty food and drinks at banquets.
18	Maintaining physical environment	It is important to maintain one's physical environment clean in order to prevent illness.
19	Managing a dangerous environment	I am quite good at managing dangerous environments, I was caught in a fire once and managed to remain calm and follow instructions.
20	Arithmetic activities	I am not very good at arithmetic activities, I have difficulty adding, subtracting, multiplying and dividing without a calculator.
21	Managing relationships with friends	Managing relationships with friends requires you to keep in touch with them and share certain parts of your life and activities.
22	Motor coordination	Your motor coordination needs to be excellent if you have to be able to play the drums.
23	Performing an activity for an extended period (psychological endurance)	I usually get very restless and distracted while performing an activity for an extended period.

24	Intellectual development and function	It is important to engage children in constructive activities for their intellectual development and function.
25	Moving around	I need to move around in the house to be able to reach the things I need.
26	Work	One needs to work in order to make a living.
27	People sharing living space	My wife and son are the people who are sharing my living space in my house.
28	Following written instructions	I have no difficulty following the written instructions that my teachers give in class.
29	Planning/organizing meals	I feel overwhelmed when I'm required to plan and organize meals as it involves coordinating shopping cooking and serving the meal.
30	Cultural activities	I enjoy cultural activities such as festivals, theater, opera etc.
31	Handling technical devices/ aids for locomotion	People need to be trained at handling technical devices for locomotion such as wheelchairs to give them more freedom of movement.
32	Communication activities	When I trained to be a teacher I had to take courses in communication activities.
33	Changing a body position	For people who are completely paralyzed it can be difficult changing a body position.
34	Following (showing interest in) events that take place outside of the direct environment	I follow events that take place outside of the direct environment by watching the news on TV and reading the newspaper.
35	Study behaviours	My study behaviours change depending on how much the subject interests me.
36	Recognizing	When I cross a friend on the street who I recognize I usually greet him.
37	Written communication	Written communication such as letters are very important for business transactions.
38	Managing general psychological demands	I have difficulties managing general psychological demands at times and feel under pressure and stress.
39	Taking care of pets/ domestic animals	I take care of my pet cat by feeding it regularly, allowing it to exercise and taking it to the doctor for its regular check ups.
40	Communication content	I should pay attention, while speaking to people, not only about the communication content but also how I say things.
41	Activities related to fulfilling of financial obligations and services	I always fulfill my financial obligations, all my taxes and bills are always paid on time.
42	Maintaining a body position	I have difficulty maintaining a body position for a length of time, after a few minutes I get restless and I feel like moving around.

43	Cooking, baking, frying solids	When cooking baking and frying solid foods, one must be careful not to overcook or burn it.
44	Conversation processes and structure	When we speak to each other, our interactions are shaped by the conversation processes and structure.
45	Abilities relating to learning and communication	Reading, writing, arithmetic, giving and taking messages build the foundations for our abilities relating to learning and communication.
46	Taking care of meals	Taking care of meals involves shopping, as well as cooking and preparing meals.
47	Dating and forming relationship	Some people have trouble dating and forming relationships because they are too shy to open up to the person they are attracted to.
48	Energy and drive	My energy and drive is what keeps me from starving, otherwise I would forget to eat.
49	Religious activities	Traditional religious activities are a time to bring families and communities with common beliefs together.
50	Psychomotor activity	When one is depressed one feels slowed down and one's psychomotor activity is decreased.
51	Handling body attached technical aids	It is really remarkable what people can really do once they have become good at handling body attached technical aids such as calipers and artificial limbs.
52	Keeping rules, abiding by decisions	Sometimes, children have difficulty keeping rules or abiding by decisions, they tend to be disobedient and rebellious.
53	Sexual functions	Sex education for adolescents is aimed at making them more aware and in touch with their sexual functions.
54	Washing oneself	I like to wash myself every morning, so that I feel clean and fresh.
55	Following verbal instructions	Following verbal instructions over the telephone can be difficult if I am not familiar with the subject matter.
56	Education	Good education helps a person to learn well and lays a good foundation for the future.
57	Language	Using foul language is something people do when upset or angry.
58	Work acquisition and retention behaviours	To succeed in one's career it is important to have the right kind of work acquisition and retention behaviours.
59	Performing consensual sexual acts	The right approach and care in performing consensual sexual acts is important for a healthy relationship.
60	Procurement and care of necessities	Persons who have a low intelligence may need help in the procurement and care of necessities of everyday life.

61	Responding to conversational cues	Responding to conversational cues is necessary to maintain an interesting conversation.
62	Taking care of household or family members	Much of my time as a housewife is spent taking care of the household or family members.
63	Monitoring and evaluating of performance of activities, tasks	Monitoring and evaluating the performance of activities and tasks helps us learn from our mistakes and do better next time.
64	Managing personal behaviour	In my relations with others I am generally careful in managing my personal behaviour and keep my mood and impulses under check.
65	Using public transport	Using public transport such as buses (or trains) can be quite a challenge at rush hour.
66	Responding to dangers	Children and old people need looking after as they may not be quick in responding to dangers.
67	Illness	I told the doctor that I caught this illness while I was travelling.

PART 2

CULTURE-SPECIFIC FINDINGS FROM THE CAR STUDY

Introduction

The chapters in this part systematically set out the findings of the CAR study in 15 CAR study sites around the world. The considerable effort put into the CAR study by these centres made the study possible and produced invaluable data, both for the revision of the ICIDH-2 and for the WHO-NIH joint project. It is anticipated that the results reported here will set the standard for cross-cultural research in disability, and will be of immense value to future researchers.

For comparability, each centre report is structured similarly. Opening with a summary of the results, the report then gives a brief introduction to the geography, demography and social situation of the area the centre represents, with an emphasis on the condition of persons with disabilities associated with physical and ADM health conditions. This is followed by a brief description of the implementation of the CAR methods, including a discussion of sampling issues. Then, in the bulk of the report, each centre summarizes their results, by methodology. The report concludes with a discussion that highlights the salient aspects of their research and its significance for disability classification and epidemiology.

Chapter 4
Cambodia

Ritu Sadana, Sisokhom Sek, and Hourn Kruy Kim[*]

Highlights from CAR study in Cambodia

- In Cambodia, between 250,000 and 450,000 of the population of 10.7 million (roughly 2–4%) experience serious physical or mental impairments or disabilities.

- Outside the capital city, only limited governmental and nongovernmental support is available for most people, even with serious disabilities, in terms of both cash subsidies and access to rehabilitation or treatment programmes.

- Individuals with disabilities are discriminated against partly because disabilities are viewed as punishments due to bad moral behaviour in a previous life.

- Individuals with disabilities want to regain their dignity through improved income-earning opportunities.

- Gender, geographical location, and availability of family support affects a person's experience of disability.

- Further discussion of the translation of ideas, not simply terms, is needed before an appropriate translation of the ICIDH-2 can be completed in Khmer.

---

[*] Harvard School of Public Health, Boston, MA, USA (Sadana); Deputy Head of the Department of Psychology, University of Phnom Penh (Sek); Lecturer in Department of Psychology, University of Phnom Penh (Kim).

Introduction

Phnom Penh

After 25 years of war and civil strife, the Royal Government of Cambodia is making a gradual transition to a post-conflict democracy. Khmers form 95% of the country's population of 10.7 million, while ethnic Chinese, Vietnamese, Cham (Muslims) and hill tribes comprise the remaining 5%, making Cambodia the most ethnically homogenous country in South-East Asia. Almost all Cambodians identify themselves as Theravada Buddhists. Rice is the principal crop while tropical rain forest timber is the most important natural resource. Cambodia has a tropical monsoon climate. Phnom Penh, the capital city, has over 800,000 inhabitants. The main site for the data gathered in the CAR study, it is located in the south of the country at the confluence of the Mekong and Tonle Sap rivers, some 150 km north of the Vietnamese border.

With minimal infrastructure and an annual per capita gross national product estimated at less that US$ 300, the country is classified as one of the least developed in the world. The average monthly household income in rural areas (US$ 48) is approximately one-fourth of that in Phnom Penh (US$ 196) (Asian Development Bank 1995; 1997 World Bank 1996). Although all the data for this study were collected in Phnom Penh, many of the participants originated from rural areas of the country and came to the capital to seek services.

Factors contributing to impairments and disabilities in Cambodia

Because of the high density of anti-personnel landmines found throughout the country (estimated at 4–6 million), approximately 150–200 individuals undergo traumatic amputations each month. Although de-mining activities are under way, these are extremely slow: at the current rate of clearance, it will take about 175 years for villagers to reclaim the agricultural land and forests currently mined.

Several qualitative studies point to the connection between physical disabilities and detrimental mental health status (Cambodian Trust 1995). In the Khmer world-view, individuals who are missing limbs or suffer from severe physical disabilities are incomplete and their physical status is thought to reflect bad actions during their previous life. These individuals are stigmatized and are often excluded from entering monasteries or attending other religious or social activities that form the basis of community life and support in Cambodia. As a result, individuals with disabilities who lack both family support and working or income-earning skills are considered the most socially and economically vulnerable in Cambodia. Children with disabilities are also especially vulnerable, as few are accepted by schools and peers.

In Cambodia, as in many developing countries, poverty and disability are associated, both as causes of disability and barriers to rehabilitation and social or environmental participation. Access to education, health services and employment opportunities for people with disabilities is limited, particularly for individuals with mental disabilities, yet these obstacles are also faced by many Cambodians simply because they live and work in rural areas. Competing demands and cultural traditions appear to limit the social and political will to mitigate the stigma attached to individuals with disabilities.

Epidemiology and support structure

Although no national population-based statistics on impairment or disability are yet available in Cambodia, either for Phnom Penh alone or for the country's more than 20 rural provinces, it is estimated that between 2% and 4% (250,000 to 450,000 people) out of the population of 10.7 million experience serious physical or mental disabilities. This proportion of severe disabilities is reportedly one of the highest in the world. In 1996, amputations and blindness each made up 20% of the total physical and mental disabilities recorded in eight major provinces; disabilities cause by polio and hearing/speech impairments each accounted for an additional 15% of the total, and paraplegia or quadriplegia, mental illness, and disabilities caused by a range of other conditions, including leprosy, each accounted for a further 10% (Handicap International 1997). Only mental illnesses of a more severe nature are included in these estimates.

Furthermore, more than 20% of all people with disabilities are children under the age of 18. Among children, polio is the major cause of physical disability, followed by visual and hearing impairments (Ministry of Social Affairs, Labour and Veteran Affairs 1995). The special needs and experiences of children were not covered in this study, but would merit separate investigation.

The Cambodian disability support structure consists of: (1) limited official governmental cash benefits or pensions that are in practice restricted to military personnel or their families; (2) nongovernmental support to individuals provided by national and international NGOs offering training, rehabilitation or counselling services for mental and physical disabilities only; and (3) family support, which is still considered the most important factor in mitigating the negative consequences of all types of disabilities in Cambodia.

Methods

Instruments

The Cambodian site completed almost all the basic and recommended components of the CAR study, including linguistic analysis, the centre description, focus groups, key informant interviews, item evaluation (concept mapping matrix), and the ranking exercise. The pile sorting was deemed not necessary and the key informant interviews were shortened in light of the analysis of other participating sites' findings, as suggested by the WHO Team. All CAR activities took place between August and November 1997.

Sample and basic methods

Linguistic analysis

The linguistic analysis of ICIDH terminology specifically used in the item evaluation and concept mapping included forward and backward translations, together with discussions to reconcile Cambodian concepts with Western terms. This analysis was carried out by a team of three urban, bilingual Cambodians specializing in public health, physical disabilities and mental disabilities.

Centre description

The centre description was completed in consultation with the head of the Cambodian Disabled People's Organization, a self-help, self-representation and cross-disability organization located in Phnom Penh. This national organization is one of two self-help groups that offer advocacy, training facilities and referral to services for individuals with disabilities.

Focus groups

Two focus groups were conducted to provide a Cambodian perspective on forms and expressions of stigma, social and environmental conditions, assessment of the ICIDH disablement model, and the identification of appropriate assessment domains for a disability assessment instrument. A balanced representation of men and women was achieved for the two groups. Group I comprised individuals with physical disabilities (N=8) and group II comprised management and field staff (N=9).

The mean age of participants in group I was 28; only 40% of them reported that they could read easily. The mean age in group II was 31; 65% of the staff were directly involved in social or field work and 75% had a physical disability themselves. Both group discussions were held at the National Rehabilitation Centre at Wat Than, Phnom Penh. This centre receives governmental support as well as support from an international NGO.

Focus groups were held in Khmer and lasted about 2 hours. The discussions were tape-recorded, transcribed verbatim, and then translated verbatim into English. Analysis and summaries are based on the English translations, with references to quotes from the original Khmer transcriptions.

Key informant interviews

Seventeen individuals were recruited for the key informant interviews and self-administered questionnaire, covering stigma and shame associated with different types of physical and mental disabilities and substance abuse (interviewer-assisted portion), as well as the item evaluation of 50 terms used in the draft ICIDH-2 and/or concepts relevant to the disability assessment instrument, and the ranking exercise of 17 different physical, mental or other less than perfect health states (self-administered portion). Both portions of the key informant interviews were carried out in Khmer and took place at the participant's office, with interviewers taking detailed notes. The entire process lasted approximately 3 hours. All qualitative responses were translated verbatim into English.

All of the key informants worked in international or national organizations addressing disabilities, with 40% being case workers, 35% teachers or trainers, and the remaining 25% working in the management of disability programmes. A full 90% currently worked in the area of physical disabilities, while 20% currently or had previously worked in the area of mental disabilities. No one worked in the area of alcohol or substance abuse, reflecting the almost total non-existence of programmes specifically targeting this group of individuals in Cambodia. Women made up 35% of the key informants, and men 65%. The average age of key informants was 33.5 years.

Procedure

The primary CAR research team in Cambodia consisted of two lecturers from the Department of Psychology, University of Phnom Penh, one social researcher experienced in physical disabilities from Cambodian Researchers for Development (a local research organization), and one international public health specialist with experience in Cambodia, who provided methodological and report writing guidance.

All individuals recruited to participate were informed of the study's general objectives and freely consented to participate before the interviews or discussions began. At the end of the interview, nonprofessional participants were offered 2000 riels-about 75 US cents to compensate for the time spent on the interview. All participants were offered refreshments. None of the participants knew in advance that they would be offered a small payment for their participation.

At the end of the interview, nonprofessional participants were provided with information on where to obtain local treatment or rehabilitation services offered by existing governmental or NGO services in the Phnom Penh area. Rehabilitation, treatment and patient group organizations that participated in the study have each received copies of all reports written so far.

Results

The results from the linguistic analysis and centre description on disability have been integrated throughout the contents of this report. Selected results from the focus groups, key informant interviews, item evaluation and ranking exercises follow.

Focus group discussions

Both groups agreed in general that individuals without disabilities evaluate and judge those with impairments or disabilities very negatively. This judgement is based not only on an individual's current physical or mental status, but also on the belief that bad moral behaviour (in a previous life) is the underlying cause of the impairment and its subsequent consequences. The burden of these negative, deterministic attitudes limits the accepted place and entitlement to opportunities that individuals with impairments have within Cambodian society and directly contributes to the shame expressed by those with impairments.

Public attitudes and misconceptions

From the perspective of those with impairments and disabilities, the general population fails to understand the true life experiences of those with impairments. Although caring, sympathetic and non-judgemental individuals exist, they seem to be the exception rather than the norm. Group participants discussed the general attitudes and misconceptions held by those without disabilities that need to be redressed through education and improved knowledge. Some of these are discussed below.

- Lack of understanding. Several participants discussed their feeling that individuals without impairments do not understand their experience. For example, one man with a below-the-knee amputation stated: "Normal people never know about our suffering ... they only look at us with a different way of thinking ... they look down on us." Another man – a polio victim – in the same group added: "People with handicaps have the same desires as normal people ... but they do not know it!"

- Begging as the main source of income. Almost all participants described the fact that individuals without impairments consider that begging is one of the only options available to those with physical disabilities. More specifically, it is assumed that those with impairments must rely on other people's pity. Several related their experiences at the market, where people treated them as beggars even if they were not begging. One woman summarized the group experience and the factors that contribute to lower self-esteem: "Even if I have money or a job, at the market people assume we are beggars. People sometimes give me money and this makes me feel bad." A man continued: "Some people with handicaps are beggars but ... it's not all people with handicaps who are beggars. But others evaluate us the same, always connecting people with handicaps with beggars."

- All individuals with disabilities are morally at fault. All participants discussed the problem that those without impairments lump together all impairments and disabilities into one category, regardless of the particular individual, his or her moral traits or character, unique capabilities, or individual personality. They argue that there are morally good individuals with impairments who are sometimes confused with the "bad ones." "Bad ones" include those who are lazy, drink alcohol, or who are angry all of the time. Most individuals in group I discussed the way they are always trying to prove to others that they are morally good (and thus do not necessarily deserve the impairment that they experience, within the Khmer world view of causation of disability). A man and a woman in group I summarized good character as "being gentle and sweet, motivated to work, showing willingness, trying to help him/herself, having hope and believing in him/herself." Others added that "those who make a living by themselves, who can help other people, who respect old age and respect their neighbour" also illustrate good moral behaviour. Such behaviour, reflecting social order and individual discipline, is highly valued in Cambodia.

- The consequences of bad moral behaviour include exclusion from social activities and normal roles, which is exactly what most individuals with physical disabilities face. An individual who is born with an impairment or who later suffers from an accident or health problem that causes an impairment is not seen as a complete human being, and being born incomplete is commonly explained as the result of bad deeds committed in a previous life. Even though many with impairments do not necessarily think they deserve their condition, the common values offer an explanation: a male staff member who has polio stated: "I think my body became like this because of my previous life ... I might have done bad actions." A woman in group I explained: "We don't want to be with handicaps, but if we think about our destiny, maybe we have committed demerits in our previous life, so in this life we have handicaps."

- People with disabilities feel insulted and shamed. Several participants recounted that in public they often face verbal insults. These include extremely pejorative terms including *kam-bot* or *kam-bak,* meaning "dismembered amputee," or "torn off, broken beggar." For women, the term *mi ankot* is often used, also extremely pejorative, meaning a female who is as useless as a log (reflecting the analogy of the body to a tree). Others mentioned that children as well as adults may imitate their disability, such as difficulty in walking. One woman staff member with polio said: "When people with disabilities live in the community, there are only a few of them, so when they go out, they feel a lot of shame ... because they are made to feel that 'normal' people have more ability ... and when they do go out, others use derogatory language or imitate them."

- Better educated individuals who do not have impairments or disabilities are encouraging. A few individuals talked about meeting some individuals who have "better education, better understanding" who tend to encourage individuals with impairments. One woman summed up by saying that these "persons with a better understanding, a good education, do not look down on a person who has had polio ... they encourage us and feel pity." A woman with a below-the-knee amputation said that: "when we behave well, people admire us; for example, now I have a job, have a good salary, and I can feed myself ... people with two legs and two arms look at me and can admire me." However, many agreed that few people try to encourage individuals with disabilities. A man with an above-the-knee amputation stated: "Most people wonder and ask 'how can you survive?'" Another woman added: "Some normal people evaluate us on the base of our capacity and behaviour, but their attitude is usually very judgemental, very negative."

• Mental impairments and bad moral behaviour are most heavily stigmatized. Most agreed that individuals with mental impairments and persons with physical impairments who also drink, gamble, sleep on the streets or visit prostitutes experience the most severe social stigma. One woman in group I summarized: "It depends on the character of the person . . . they [those without impairments] hate us if we behave badly." For the latter group, this indicates bad moral behaviour in this life as well. Individuals with mental impairments, especially *ckeut,* the Khmer concept for active psychosis, are particularly ostracized or exploited. Women who have both physical and mental impairments are most vulnerable; many agreed that "sometimes men rape them." In general, women who display bad moral behaviour are evaluated more negatively than men. Two women in group I summed this up: "In Cambodia, when women act wrongly, others are quick to look down on them. As for men who are bad, however, it is considered more normal for them to drink, for example, and then no one looks down on them as much."

Obstacles and barriers

In both groups, the distinction between activity and participation issues was clearly articulated through the detailed examples based on lived experiences, Khmer proverbs and folk tales, that are described in the full Cambodian report. In summary, the various obstacles and barriers preventing full participation are most serious for the 85% of the population living in rural areas, those with mental disabilities or substance abuse problems, and for women, and include the following problems:

• Social/community participation obstacles that often reinforce feelings of shame and isolation. Individuals mentioned that although personal attitudes and character are important, the social response is a very powerful negative barrier to participation and being accepted in the community. A woman noted: "People who don't know us look down on us – they say they cannot do anything ... when we go to the ceremony we think that we can share happiness with them (those without disabilities) but at that moment these people treat us strangely ... so we understand, that's the way they look down on us, we can see their negative attitude and its influence on us." Several examples clearly showed how the experience of negative social interaction led to shame. Most individuals noted that they were least comfortable with strangers or strange situations. A male staff member who had

had polio related: "When I come to meetings, when I meet people I know ... I feel good ... no shame. If I go outside, into another community, I feel bad sometimes." Another staff member added: "For those living at the centre, they live with people who are similar and it's okay ... when they go back to their own village, they will again experience some bad feelings but, I hope not as strong as before they came to the centre."

Many individuals and staff mentioned that shame restricts social interaction, by reducing people's motivation to go outside their dwelling or household. Others said that neighbours also make comments on their disability, increasing their disappointment with themselves. A few participants noted that even "family members still blame us, just as society does." A woman noted that her family "didn't want me to go on a picnics with them, but to stay at home." A few women in both groups remarked that the social stigma is greater for women with physical disabilities than for men. Women provided some general impressions, for example: "A man with a disability can take on a pretty wife who has two good legs and arms, but if a woman is missing a leg, she can not have a 'complete' man to love her."

- Educational opportunity limitations, which contribute to the negative downward spiral of disability, poor education, and dependence on others for survival. Many participants commented that they had fewer opportunities for education, especially if they had had their impairment from birth or during childhood. One woman described the interaction between disability and poor education. As she said: "As we have disabilities, we do lack some capacity, yet we are also less educated, so when we study something, it is difficult for us to understand quickly ... we try but it's impossible ... even at this centre [Wat Than] they are most likely to help those who already have some education."

- Economic participation barriers in terms of real earnings and jobs held, rather than the availability of training or rehabilitation services. Many participants said that even with appropriate skills, they are unable to find jobs or earn a living. Another woman in group I noted: "Even if we have good sewing skills , we have disabilities, so we cannot earn money like a dress-maker who has no impairment, and so we still suffer." Sometimes these obstacles to participation are based on the poor match between the jobs available, particularly in rural areas, and the skills that individuals possess. In the countryside, the rice-based agriculture demands that men plough and women tend the fields, particularly during the transplanting season. Therefore, individuals who cannot do this particularly strenuous physical work are generally viewed as dependent on those who take part in rice production.

Self-perception and attitudes to people without disabilities

Both groups discussed their own self-perception and their attitudes towards those without impairments or disabilities:

• Self-perception. Individuals pointed out that they have the same ideas, feelings and desires as those without disabilities; however, participants discussed the following main differences between them and those without impairments or disabilities:

Physical disabilities. Individuals in both groups discussed different types of physical disabilities in terms of limitations in the range of work, scope of activities and amount of energy, as well as general difficulties in mobility, walking, sleeping, standing and sitting. One man with an above-the-knee amputation explained: "I use an artificial leg but it is difficult for me to do hard work, such as carry water or other heavy things. I can't walk or run fast. Before, I could do everything, but now I only do light work, and I do it slowly." A man who had had polio noted: "I don't know how to do hard physical work, as I have had polio since I was born."

Reduced ability to find solutions to general problems because of the physical and psychological impact of impairment. Participants repeated two Khmer proverbs that illustrate how physical impairments are connected to problem-solving: *"Muc min chrev tev min craay,"* meaning literally "Diving in water not deep enough and not going far enough," which means "Thinking but not finding the appropriate solution." The frustration of many participants was summed up in another proverb: "Having theory but no practice" meaning "Impossible to really do something."

Some individuals in both groups had physical impairments and they discussed how this affected emotions and psychology. One man with an above-the-knee amputation said: "My mind doesn't work well sometimes … it cannot catch information as quickly as someone who is without physical disabilities, someone normal." Another man who had had polio noted: "I'm very angry and blame myself when I do something slowly." Most participants mentioned that when they feel inadequate, they have lower self-esteem and self-confidence: as one woman who is height-impaired noted: "Most are disappointed with themselves."

Must be better morally than others. All participants said that their actions and attitudes must be morally and socially good, potentially as a way to show others that they deserve to be respected actively, rather than simply to be offered pity by others. As mentioned, being patient, controlling one's temper and respecting neighbours and the elderly illustrate good moral behaviour. Controlling anger is also viewed as a prerequisite to absorbing new information and learning new skills.

- Attitudes towards people with no apparent disabilities. Both men and women said that individuals without disabilities are "pretty, beautiful." These characteristics are the most commonly mentioned, and are also the most commonly discussed signs of positive health in Cambodia in general. Several also commented that those without disabilities "have the capacity for a range of activities and work," not surprisingly the positive side of the limitations they experience. As a result, the overall life situation of those without impairments or disabilities is "very different." Basic necessities such as food, shelter and appropriate clothing appear to be less of a problem for those without disabilities. One woman who had had polio summed up the difference: "I want it [a minimum standard of living], but it's impossible."

Areas for improvement

Both groups agreed on key areas for improvement, including:

- Earn income. The highest priority is to obtain a job and earn sufficient income to reduce dependence on others and avoid negative social judgements, which in turn would improve self-confidence. A woman with a below-the-knee amputation from a land-mine accident summed up, "If people with disabilities join the work force, we will not have problems because we can understand and put trust in ourselves. With a job, we can join the community. They [people without disabilities] will accept us, we can then join festivals and go to the pagoda."
- Job placement. Further support is needed for job placement appropriate to the capacity of the individual, underscoring that training alone is not enough to ensure jobs because of the heavy discrimination in the job sector.
- Improve image. There is also a need for stronger solidarity among individuals with disabilities, which would emphasize and promote the positive qualities of each individual.

In addition, not all people with injuries, particularly in rural areas, receive the entitlements that are due to them. Villagers are sometimes tricked into selling their disability pension to unscrupulous individuals, sometimes for US$20 or US$50. Then these individuals will collect the benefit directly from the Government, potentially receiving 10 or 20 what they have paid to the villager. Participants added that government support is often inappropriate and consists more of symbolic gestures by politicians rather than substantial support towards increasing their autonomy or self-reliance. Appropriate support would not necessarily include food or clothing simply given away, but might involve providing access to rice fields, or some form of support that is more sustainable. Most agreed with one man's estimate that "out of 100 people who need help, maybe only 12 or sometimes no one gets support ... and people in the rural areas only get support by chance." Given that 85% of the population lives in rural areas, this is a concern for many Cambodians. Yet a few added: "In urban areas, among those with disabilities ... most of them get a little support, but not from the Government."

Implications for an assessment instrument

The two groups were asked which topics, experiences or concerns of individuals with impairments or disabilities would be most useful to assess to understand their situation and offer them appropriate assistance. Their spontaneous responses are summarized in Table 1:

Table 1. Comparison of key concerns/important domains for assessment, Cambodia, 1997

I. Individuals with impairments/ disabilities	II. Staff (many with impairments/disabilities)
1. Autonomy, including economic activity and decision-making	1. Good health (positive signs)
2. Mobility	2. Job/ability to be independent financially
3. Self-perception	3. Ability to absorb and use knowledge
4. Social impact and exclusion from "normal life"	4. Social recognition and integration
5. Psychological impact	5. Good moral actions and solidarity between those who have impairments and those who do not
6. Economic impact (resulting from a combination: of factors 1–5 listed above) including access to enough food, decent clothing, clean dwelling	6. Dwelling/decent housing
	7. Physical and mental capacity and ability
	8. Ability to contribute views and ideas
	9. Technical or other type of skill (as distinct from having a job)

Both groups referred to the importance of assessing general living standards, physical abilities, ability to contribute ideas or make decisions, and social integration. Group I, composed only of individuals with impairments or disabilities, also stressed the assessment of self-perception and psychological aspects of the individual, as a key to understanding their experience. Staff members, in group II, stressed that general positive health and the skills individuals possess should also be assessed, as these are particularly important in determining what practical types of assistance can be provided to individuals with impairments or disabilities.

After the spontaneous discussion, the six domains selected by the WHO working group (understanding the world around you, moving and getting around, life activities, self-care, getting along with people, and participation in society) were discussed and presented to group II comprising staff members. Participants in this group responded that the six points were directly related to the nine points they proposed for assessment (see table 1). Except for commenting on the need to separate citizenship from economic life, participants seemed hesitant to critique or directly alter the six domains presented. Only one woman ventured: "We seemed to add important points for Cambodia."

Key informant interviews: evaluation of stigma and shame

Quantitative stigma ratings

Of the 18 health conditions presented, the four least stigmatizing conditions (rated from 3 to 6 out of 10) were: inability to read, cannot keep a job, borderline intelligence and obesity. The five most stigmatizing conditions (rated either 9 or 10 out of 10) were: HIV-positivity, drug addiction, alcoholism, leprosy, and facial disfigurement.

Qualitative understanding of the experience of living with four distinct, representative disabilities

Social norms were discussed in detail for each of the following four disabilities: difficulty walking or getting around; bothered by strange thoughts; born with low intelligence; and uncontrolled drinking of alcohol. The following dimensions were discussed with a summary of the results in Table 2:

- Labelling – negative social recognition and labelling
- Disability – serious signs and impact on daily activities
- Economic role – barrier to participate in productive work
- Social role – barrier to getting married and having a family
- Official support – length of time before entitlement to social assistance and perceived right to benefits
- Early life – differences in social perception if disability was experienced from birth or early childhood, if applicable)

The in-depth key informant interviews (and summary table above) show that physical disabilities, and to a greater degree mental disabilities, are quite highly stigmatized in a variety of ways in Cambodia. However, individuals born with lower intelligence are less likely to be labelled as such and also suffer from fewer barrier to social and economic participation. This reflec-

Table 2. Evaluation of stigma and shame with four disabilities in various dimensions, Cambodia, 1997

	Difficulty getting around	Having strange thoughts	Low IQ	Alcohol problem
Labelling	high	high	medium	medium
Disability	high	high	medium	medium
Economic role	medium	medium	low	high
Social role	high	high	medium	high
Official support	low	medium	medium	high
Early life	low	medium	low	—

tion is also confirmed in the low ranking of disability attached to mild mental retardation, noted below.

Although individuals with alcohol problems may be less likely to be perceived as having disabilities or activity limitations, they are more likely to experience negative social judgements. The social consensus is that these individuals have the greatest personal responsibility for their disability, and are least likely to benefit from services or support.

Key informant interviews: item evaluation/concept mapping exercise

Concept mapping exercises indicated that the following items require further clarification:

- *Acquiring and applying knowledge* (need to specify type of education or norm);
- *Leisure* (conceptually absent from many peoples' lives);
- *Managing a dangerous environment* ("surviving in a dangerous environment" preferred);
- *Citizenship* (political freedom and democracy in terms of governmental institutions are at an early stage);
- *Maintaining close relationships* (the Khmer concept of relationships is based on both parties, and differs if within a couple, in the family or between relatives, among friends or in community, or patron-client relationships);
- *Understanding the meaning of written language* ("being able to read" preferred);
- *School-related behaviours;*
- *Sexual functioning;*

- *Methods of breathing/respiration;*
- *Immunological functions;*
- *Muscular force;*
- *Caring for own well-being;*
- *Insight.*

The items considered most problematic were those that are most conceptual, abstract, or rooted in English idiomatic expressions, and therefore also difficult to translate into non-technical Khmer language, such as "insight." However, almost all items were judged as not capable of being used equally among different groups in Cambodia, to some degree reflecting the linguistic structure of the most common Cambodian language, Khmer, where the relationship between speakers alters the terminology used. The key informants interpreted this evaluation question strictly, and upon further probing noted that as long as the proper subject, verb and object reflecting the relationship and sensitivity of the person being addressed were also attached to each concept, most items would be appropriate.

Key informant interviews: rank ordering of disability

On a scale where 1 was the most disabling condition and 17 the least disabling, the four most severely disabling conditions (average ranks between 3.5 and 4.9) were: quadriplegia, HIV-positivity, active psychosis and total blindness. The five very disabling conditions (average ranks between 7.4 and 9.6) were: paraplegia, dementia, drug dependence, total deafness and alcoholism. The four moderately disabling conditions (average ranks between 10.2 and 11.4) were: below-the-knee amputation, major depression, severe migraines, and vitiligo on face. The least disabling conditions (average ranks between 12.1 and 14) of the 17 health states ranked were: incontinence, infertility, mild mental retardation, and rheumatoid arthritis.

Although participants were requested to factor in participation problems, most weighted functional or psychological disability greatest in their evaluation. It is important to note that the listing above does not represent the relative value that individuals place on different conditions, but only their rank order within the 17 conditions presented. These rankings do not provide ordinal or ratio values among health states.

It is surprising to note, in contrast to the key informants, that among individuals with disabilities (who also completed this exercise, first individually and then as a group) one of the conditions remained unranked: below-the-knee amputation. This group did not wish to rank this condition, possibly because about half of this group had this impairment. Although the group discussion was rich on this topic, individuals did not seem to want to place their personal experiences in a ranking with other conditions they were less familiar with.

Conclusion

Better awareness and understanding of the needs of individuals with disabilities is greatly needed in Cambodia. This belief is held by both individuals with disabilities and professionals working in this sector.

The CAR study results indicated that the cross-cultural saliency of a model describing disabilities/activity limitations on the one hand, and participation restrictions/social or economic consequences on the other, is applicable to the Cambodian context. However, the actual levels, forms and expressions of activity limitations and participation barriers differ, depending on the type of disability and a variety of socio-demographic characteristics.

Additional findings are:

- Although there may be some parity between physical and mental health disabilities may exist, many of the individuals with physical disabilities had had more time to adjust or adapt to the physical impairment or disability, while individuals interviewed with psychological or other mental health disabilities were often seeking treatment for the first time, or currently under treatment. Thus, some assessment of the individual's adaptation to the problem is required.

- Other demographic variables were found to be important, in particular gender, geographical location, and availability of family support.

- Governmental support is limited for people even with serious disabilities; this is so within the wider context of a post-conflict society that is re-building governmental, religious and civil institutions and developing its commitment to human rights.

- Further discussion of the translation of ideas, not simply words, is needed before an appropriate translation of the ICIDH-2 is completed in Khmer.

- For the assessment instrument, the addition of other topics or domains, such as basic necessities, psychological experience, and job placement support, is very important and these topics are not specifically addressed in the first version of the questionnaire. The additions would make the assessment instrument and the ICIDH-2 model more suitable for use in practice in Cambodia.

These findings and conclusions are based on a limited sample of participants and should not be generalized to all individuals with disabilities in Cambodia, particularly individuals from different ethnic or religious backgrounds.

Acknowledgements

The research team would like to thank all organizations and individuals involved in the CAR study in Cambodia, including Handicap International, the National Centre for Rehabilitation at Wat Than, the Cambodian People's Disabled Organizations, and especially all the individuals who participated in the interviews. The Cambodian research team included: Mrs Hema Nhong, Head of the Department of Psychology, University of Phnom Penh; Mrs Youthea Sdeoun Van, researcher, Cambodian Researchers for Development; and Dr Sokuntea Sau Margain, formerly in charge of maternal and child health services in Kandal Province. Mrs Sek and Mrs Kruy Kim have contributed significantly to the subsequent quantitative field testing of the revised WHO Disability Assessment Schedule (WHODAS II) pilot tests.

Chapter 5
Canada – Toronto

*Angela Paglia, Jürgen Rehm, and Robin Room**

Highlights from CAR study in Ontario, Canada

- There is a lack of parity between physical and mental health conditions in terms of public opinion.
- Disability is often judged and evaluated in the context of underlying causes.
- The concept of "Participation" as a key dimension in ICIDH-2 is gradually gaining acceptance in Canada.
- Long-term impairments are still the prototype of publicly accepted disabilities.
- Disabilities referring to sexual functioning and self-care are seen as culturally sensitive in Canada.

Disabilities in Ontario

This centre report is based on data gathered in Ontario, which has often been described as being closest to the Canadian average in many respects. Canada has a total population of 28.8 million. Ontario, the most populous province, has about 10.7 million residents; 12% of them are over 65 years of age, 67% are aged 15–64, and 21% are under 15 years of age. Some 13% of the Canadian population aged 15–64 reports having a disability (Statistics Canada 1993).

* Centre for Addiction and Mental Health, Addition Research Foundation Division, Toronto, Ontario, Canada (Paglia, Rehm, Room); Centre for Social Research on Alcohol and Drugs, Sveåplan, Stockholm University, Stockholm, Sweden (Room).

The Canadian disability support structure, which is applicable in Ontario, consists of three basic systems. Each province has a *workers' compensation system,* financed by workplace taxes, which covers income and rehabilitation services for work-related injuries or illnesses. A *national pension plan* financed from wage-related taxes pays disability benefits to those who have been in the workforce who experience severe and permanent disabilities; partial and temporary disabilities are not covered. *Social assistance (welfare)* provides support for those who do not qualify under the other two systems. Provincially run, but with half the financing from the federal Government, until recently, this system has covered the "disabled," the "severely handicapped," and the "permanently unemployable." Most people with a mental disability fall into this system.

Ontario is now implementing sweeping changes to the disability support system. A new disability support programme was legislated in 1997. This is separate from the general social support ("welfare") system, which has been reoriented to helping those receiving welfare to become and stay employed. As finally enacted, the new legislation specifically excludes from disability support those with alcohol or drug dependence, but with no other impairment. (As originally introduced, the exclusion would have been more severe, excluding any impairment caused by drinking or non-prescribed drug use.)

The Canadian disability support system is criticized for its distinctions by cause of the disability, so that people with similar needs often receive different compensation. In particular, disabilities from accidents generally receive more support than those that are congenital or arise from illness. There is also criticism of the inefficiency of overlapping systems, each with its own set of eligibility criteria, procedures, and benefit levels.

Methods

Instruments

The Canadian site completed all basic components of the CAR study (the focus groups and linguistic analysis were not conducted): (1) key informant interviews, followed by the self-administered questionnaire; (2) pile sorting; and (3) concept mapping techniques.

The Canadian centre chose an additional 10 concepts to be included in the concept mapping matrix: initiating conversation; terminating conversation; structure of the frontal lobe; understanding general symbols; cognition and learning activities; telecommunication; taste; transport of food; movement pattern in walking; friends and close acquaintances.

Sample

Fifteen subjects were recruited for the key informant interviews and self-administered questionnaire. The sample consisted of three medical professionals; three allied health professionals; three policy-makers or opinion leaders; three ADM (alcohol, drug and mental) health consumers or care-givers; and three physical health consumers or care-givers.

The mean age of the key informant sample was 40.3 (SD=13.5). Twelve (80%) subjects were female, and three (20%) were male. Ten reported ever working in the area of physical disabilities; 13 reported ever working in the area of mental health; and only two ever worked in the alcoho or drug field.

A second sample (N=30) completed the concept mapping and pile sort instruments. Five subjects were medical professionals in the area of physical health; 10 new medical professionals in the area of ADM health; five were physical health consumers or care-givers; and 10 were ADM health consumers/care-givers. The mean age for this sample was 41.8 years (SD=10.3). Half (15) of the sample was female. Fifteen reported ever working in the physical disabilities area; 19 in the mental health area; and 10 in the alcohol or drug area. Nine subjects reported ever having a physical disability; five reported ever having a mental disability; and 15 reported ever having an alcohol or drug problem.

Both samples were recruited between February and April 1997 in the same manner. Professionals were recruited using both focused and convenience sampling procedures. Potential subjects were faxed an invitation to participate, which included a description of the study purpose and procedures. The ADM and physical consumers and care-givers were recruited through poster advertisements placed at the site. Where the sub-sampling requirements for the two study components overlapped (e.g., medical professionals, ADM consumers), subjects were randomly assigned to one of the two.

Procedures

Professionals in both components chose either to come to the site, or to be visited by an interviewer at their place of work. All consumers and care-givers were required to come to the site; they were the only sub-sample to be paid a nominal amount for participating.

Two interviewers were used for the key informant interview and self-administered questionnaire component. Before the interview, subjects were required to sign a consent form and complete a face sheet consisting of demographic questions. The interviewer then briefly described the purpose of the study and proceeded with the interview schedule. The interviews were not tape-recorded; all answers were written by the interviewer. Following the interview, each subject completed the self-administered questionnaire. Finally, subjects completed the rank-order task.

For the concept mapping and pile sort component, each subject was first asked to sign the consent form and complete the face sheet. The researcher briefly described both instruments, provided instructions, and then left the subject to complete the tasks alone. The pile sort instrument was completed first, followed by the concept mapping matrix. The entire component lasted about 2.5 hours.

Results

Key informant interview and self-administered questionnaire

Qualitative analysis

Qualitative analysis of the interviews revealed that in colloquial Canadian language "disability" or "handicap" can simultaneously refer to issues of impairment, activity limitation, and lack of participation.

Regarding physical and mental parity and societal participation, key informants said that those with physical problems would find it easier to find employment or get married and have a family because there was less societal stigma and isolation. Those with an alcohol or heroin problem would find it easy to get a job or get married, but could not sustain either for very long.

Disabilities from birth, or caused by a road accident, were seen as deserving sympathy. However, if the accident was caused by the person's own actions (e.g., drinking and driving) then the person was seen as less deserving of any sympathy or assistance. Similarly, people with substance use problems were viewed as personally responsible for making those choices, and thus were not believed to deserve compensation.[1] However, almost all respondents indicated that treatment was necessary in such cases. A personal tragedy given as a cause for an alcohol or heroin problem would not be tolerated as an excuse for very long. A majority considered that compensation for health problems seen as worthy should commence as soon as a medical authority verifies the condition.

---

[1] Interestingly, one policy-maker – foreshadowing the legislative changes later adopted in Ontario – spoke about a changing climate in Canada in which substance abusers are increasingly considered to be "moral failures." Thus, support for them should be conditional on medical authorization and mandatory treatment

Quantitative analysis

Stigma ratings
Of the 18 health conditions presented, the three least stigmatizing conditions were being blind, being wheelchair-bound, and being unable to read. The three most stigmatizing were not taking care of one's children, drug addiction, and being homeless.

Public reactions ratings
Of the 10 conditions presented, the three that were considered to elicit most negative reactions in Canadian society were: being under the influence of drugs, being visibly drunk, and being dirty and unkempt. The least negative reactions were directed at a woman in her 8th month of pregnancy, a person in a wheelchair, and a blind person.

Rank-order of disabilities
The three conditions perceived most disabling were: active psychosis, quadriplegia, and dementia. The three least disabling conditions were: vitiligo on the face, infertility, and incontinence.

Activities
Calculations of the average rating for the likelihood that "people would be surprised if the person did this activity" across all 10 activities were made for each of the five health conditions. Results revealed the following order of conditions from being least likely to most likely to elicit surprise: person with an alcohol problem, in a wheelchair, with a heroin problem, born with low intelligence, and who hears voices.

The same calculation was made for the question "Is it likely that anyone would place restrictions or barriers on the person?" The order from least likely to most likely to face barriers was: person with an alcohol problem, with a heroin problem, in a wheelchair, born with low intelligence, and who hears voices.

Concept mapping and pile sorting

The main results from the concept mapping and pile sorting are presented in Table 1. A number of items were identified by one or more informants as needing clarification or being potentially culturally sensitive in the diverse multicultural context of Ontario.

Table 1. Problematic items and dimensions for Canada (concept mapping)

Needs clarification:
- Mobility (concept)
- Procurement and care of necessities (item)
- Community (item and concept)
- Following (showing interest in) events that take place outside the direct environment (item and concept)
- Communication content (item and concept)

Difficult to use in culture:
- Keeping appropriate physical contact, and maintenance of social space

Not useful for all age groups:
- Civic and community life
- Citizenship responsibilities
- Work
- Activities related to fulfilling of financial obligations and services
- Sexual functions
- Performing consensual sexual acts

Culturally sensitive (taboo):
- Sexual functions
- Performing consensual sexual acts
- Religious activities
- Washing oneself
- Keeping appropriate physical contact, and maintenance of social space
- Dating and forming relationships

Conclusions

Overall, the following factors were illuminated by the various components of the CAR study.

1. There is a lack of parity between physical and mental health conditions in terms of public opinion.

Generally, people with obvious physical health conditions are least likely to face social stigma in Canadian society – especially if there is no apparent link to personal responsibility – compared to those with an alcohol, drug, or mental (ADM) condition. ADM disorders were also rated as eliciting more public disapproval than physical conditions.

The key informant results revealed that people consider mental health conditions more disabling and problematic than physical or substance use problems. It was thought that gaining employment would be difficult, as would getting married and having a family. Some informants commented that the idea of someone with a mental health condition having children is frowned upon by many. Thus, full participation by those with mental disabilities is barred by societal attitudes. Interestingly, those with substance use problems are thought not to face the level of barriers to participation that are faced by those with mental disabilities (key informant interview and self-administered questionnaire data). Informants felt that this might be explained by the ease of concealment of the former.

2. Disability is often judged and evaluated in the context of underlying causes.

This statement pertains to the existing federal and provincial compensation programmes in Canada, as well as to the results of the various empirical studies. The compensation system is based not only on a concept of disability that is grounded in observable symptoms, but also on the origin of the disability. For instance, one of the three largest disability compensation systems in Canada (workers' compensation) is limited to situations in which the accident or cause is linked to the workplace. Other cause-specific programmes include federal allowances for war veterans with disabilities, provincial programme for victims of crime and those who have become disabled while assisting police efforts, and automobile insurance plans.

There are, however, "back up" systems that rely to a lesser extent on cause of disabilities. One is the Canada/Québec pension Plan. However, even this is restricted by those who have previously made wage-related contributions. The most universal system in Canada is welfare (social assistance), supporting all people who demonstrate financial need. Disability-related welfare benefits are usually higher than regular welfare payments, and the fact that disability must be established through medical assessment reflects the disease-disability link.

The importance of causation is also reflected in the key informant data. The informants interviewed reported that substance abuse was viewed as caused by the person, which meant that it would be considered not to qualify for receiving social assistance. The high social disapproval ratings for alcohol and drug abusers, in terms of stigmatization and negative public reactions, support this interpretation.

In summary, the real or perceived cause of disability determines public opinion and compensation to a considerable degree. On the other hand, there is a safety net in welfare based on more universal definitions, although there is now a specific exception for alcohol or drug addiction.

3. The concept of "Participation" as a key dimension in ICIDH-2 is gradually gaining acceptance in Canada.

Although many still see disabilities as stable characteristics of individuals, the idea that society is an important agent in either enabling or hindering "participation" of persons with certain health conditions is becoming increasingly accepted. This change has been advanced by the disability movement in North America. For example, a recent decision of the Supreme Court of Canada (*Eldridge v. British Columbia*, 1997) supports the view that enabling those with disabilities to gain full participation is society's responsibility. Specifically, the court decided that publicly-funded Medicare in the province of British Columbia should pay for sign-language translation in order to allow deaf people to participate equally in the provision of medical care. On the other hand, the results of the pile sorting and concept mapping showed that the particular items used which refer to participation are highly ambiguous and problematic on all dimensions in a Canadian context. Thus, there is at this point a considerable gap between popular views and the conceptual underpinnings of ICIDH-2.

In terms of participation, Canada seems to allow comparatively high levels of participation for persons with disabilities. However, in order to participate (e.g., to gain employment), those with alcohol or drug problems must conceal their condition, according to information from the key informant study.

4. Long-term impairments are still the prototype of publicly accepted disabilities.

Conditions such as paraplegia or blindness are considered prototypical for legal definitions as well as in the judgements of survivors and health professionals. For instance, in the Canada/Québec Pension Plan, only "severe and prolonged mental and physical disabilities" are compensated. The concepts of partial or temporary disabilities are not accepted at all in this plan. The Ontario disability support legislation recognizes disabilities that are "recurrent" as well as those that are "continuous." Compensation for disability by welfare had been restricted in Ontario to "disabled persons," the "severely handicapped" or the "permanently unemployable," again indicating that long-term, stable conditions are considered prototypical.

Implicitly, mental disabilities are sometimes excluded by current definitions, especially for temporary disabilities based on chronic relapsing conditions (e.g., alcohol dependence, depression, schizophrenia). Welfare covers some of these cases, when based on a medical diagnosis other than alcohol and drug dependence (e.g., major depression). In the new Ontario law, addiction or dependence is specifically excluded as a disability.

5. Disabilities referring to sexual functioning and self-care are seen as culturally sensitive in Canada.

In the concept mapping and the pile sorting exercises, culturally sensitive items (i.e., taboo in Canadian culture) were those referring to activities and descriptions of participation relating to sexual functioning and self-care. These items also showed a higher degree of problems with universal applicability (e.g., useful in the culture, for different age groups, both genders, different social/economic groups and ethnic/cultural minority groups).

Chapter 6
Greece

*V.G. Mavreas, M. Kontea, M. Asimaki, I. Giouzelis, E. Katsikas,
K. Kollias, E. Polyzopoulos, D. Tsiongris, and C.N. Stefanis**

Highlights from the CAR study in Greece

- There is a lack of parity in both services available and stigma between mental health disabilities and physical disabilities.
- The rank-ordering of health conditions showed that the most chronic and incurable diseases are considered most disabling.
- Mental health conditions (dementia, depression, psychotic episodes) rank among the most serious disabilities, from the perspective of both health professionals and patients.

Introduction

The Greek WHO collaborating centre for the CAR study is based at the University Mental Health Research Institute (UMHRI), which is associated with the Department of Psychiatry of the University of Athens Medical School, based at Eginition Hospital. The hospital is quite small, with 150 beds, divided between the Departments of Neurology and Psychiatry in the University Medical School. The Department of Psychiatry, apart from the inpatient wards, has an outpatient department, a day hospital, a community mental health centre serving an area with a population of 100,000 inhabitants, and three rehabilitation units for psychiatric patients. Medical (and psychiatric) care in Greece has not been decentralized yet (with the exception of the community mental health centres), although under a new law to be completed soon, mental health care will become part of the public health system. Theo-

* University of Athens Medical School, Athens, Greece.

retically, the hospital and all its units (except the community centres) take care of patients from all over the country, although the great majority come from the greater Athens area.

Greece forms the southern part of the Balkan peninsula. It has a population of 10.5 million inhabitants, according to the latest (1991) census. It is a mountainous country, with small areas of plains, the biggest of which are in central and northern Greece. This geography creates problems in communication, since the road network is not well developed. The age composition of the Greek population, according to the 1991 census, was as follows: 0–14 years, 18.6%; 15–64 years, 67.2%; 65+ years, 14.2%. The population growth rate in Greece is one of the smallest in Europe. In the period 1970–1980, the average annual growth of the population was 1% and, in 1980–1990 0.5%, the projections since 1990 are about 0.1%. This means that the population is ageing, and that the country has a demographic problem. Estimates indicate that 23.5% of the population will be over 65 years old in 2025.

Greece is included among the developed nations: the UN places it in the upper-middle-income economies. Over the past 50 years the standard of living has constantly improved. Nevertheless, Greece has the lowest wages of the European Union. Unemployment has been rising in the past five years, and has reached approximately 10% at present. This development is an expected outcome of the shift of the economy to liberalism from the social democracy model prevailing in the 1980s. A national health system was established in 1983 which provides health care coverage at all three levels. However, the situation regarding the provision of health care is rather complicated, because it is provided not only by the National Health System, but also by many insurance organizations, primarily in primary care. A second problem for comprehensive coverage of health care is the lack of decentralization of health services and a system of audit and evaluation of these services.

The Greek disability support system consists of two administrative categories, social insurance (a contributory and earnings-related system); and social assistance (a non-contributory and means-tested flat-rate system). Social insurance benefits are provided by a number of insurance organizations created chiefly by the trade unions for different occupations and supported financially by employees, employers and the State (about 50 organizations for main insurance coverage and 250 for auxiliary insurance and sickness insurance). The Institute of Social Insurance (IKA) is the biggest insurance agency. It serves the largest proportion of the population, and mainly covers employees in the private sector. The Fund of the independent free-working and Small Entrepreneurs (TEVE) predominantly covers individuals that are self employed. The Organization of Agricultural Insurance (OGA) is another large insurance organization, supported mainly by the State and special taxation which covers farmers and their families. Disability benefits are provided after reports by health specialists have been reviewed by the competent health committees. Disability pensions are based on the loss of earning power and the level of benefit tends to be proportionate to the extent of lost earnings. For 67 % disability, the disabled person receives 75% of the retirement pension (100% in the case of mental health disorders) and for 80% disability, 100% of the retirement pension. Disability percentages are determined according to diagnosis and chronicity and not after an assessment of the real level of disability. The system is very complicated because of the large number of insurance organizations and the different systems of rules and percentages followed by them (although most of them follow similar rules to those of IKA). The current tendency is to merge similar funds (e.g., IKA and TEVE) and simplify the system of benefits.

Methods

The Greek site completed all the basic components of the CAR study (with the exception of the focus groups – to be conducted with the focus groups for the WHO Disability Assessment Schedule (DAS-II) study). These included (1) linguistic analysis, (2) key informant interviews, (3) self-administered questionnaires, (4) pile sorting, and (5) concept mapping. The Greek centre chose (at random) an additional 10 concepts to be included in the concept mapping matrix. These concepts were: terminating conversation, communication, structure of the frontal lobe, interacting with other specified work-related persons, performing gross visual tasks, remembering, cognition and learning activities, appropriate storage of food, understanding spoken communications, and working independently.

Sample

Linguistic analysis

The translation into Greek was conducted by a Greek expert in psychiatric rehabilitation with a good knowledge of English and experience of working in England. In addition, comments on the translation were made by the investigators. The back-translation into English was carried out independently by two experts: a psychiatrist with a good knowledge of English and interest in linguistics, and a linguist working at the Department of English Studies in the School of Philosophy, University of Athens.

Key informant interviews and self-administered questionnaires

Fifteen subjects were recruited for the key informant interviews and self-administered questionnaires study. The sample consisted of three physicians, all with extensive experience in rehabilitation and disability; two psychiatrists and a physician in physical medicine, three other health professionals working in rehabilitation (a social worker, an occupational therapist and a physiotherapist), three patients suffering from chronic disabling disorders (two with a mental and one with a physical disorder); three relatives of patients with chronic health conditions (two with a mental and one with a physical disorder); and three policy-makers working in administration in fields related to disablement. The mean age of the sample was 44.2 years (SD=11.1). Nine of the subjects were males (40%) and 9 females (40%). Professionals had a diversity of experiences. One of the psychiatrists was an expert in psychiatric rehabilitation and the other was working at the IKA in the committees for disablement benefits. All participants were either experts in disablement, or sufferers and family members with direct or indirect experience of the consequences of health problems.

Pile sorting

Twenty-five subjects participated in this exercise (with the same subjects participating in the concept mapping study). The sample consisted of mental health professionals (psychiatrists, psychologists, social workers, occupational therapists), physical health professionals (physicians, physiotherapists), mental health patients and family members, and patients with physical health problems and their family members. Twelve of the subjects were males and 12 females, while one did not note his/her gender.

Concept mapping

Twenty-nine subjects (14 males, 14 females and one who did not note his/her gender) participated in the concept mapping study. Their mean age was 41.5 years (SD=12.4) and their average duration of education was 14.4 years (SD=5.2). The composition of the sample was similar to that of the pile sorting exercise.

Focus groups

No focus groups were held at this stage of the research. However the center plans to include the questions in the focus groups of the DAS-II study in the near future.

Procedures

Linguistic analysis

Two lists of items (provided by WHO) were given to the translator who prepared the Greek translation within two weeks. Afterwards, the main site investigator commented upon the translation, and the two final lists were given to the two back-translators, who returned the back-translations within three weeks. An annotated manuscript with the translations and back-translations was prepared by the principal investigator, after discussions with all the linguistic expert group.

Key informant interviews and self-administered questionnaires

The participants in the key informant interviews study were recruited between March and May 1997. Professionals were recruited, by use of convenient sampling procedures, from those working at rehabilitation units or other services working mainly with disabled people (e.g. private physiotherapy, committees for disability benefits). Professionals and policy-makers who participated were considered to be experts on disability, with long experience in different fields of rehabilitation, either mental or physical, or in administrative and legal aspects of disability. Patients and family members were selected by their physician (in psychiatry or physical medicine). The main criterion for eligibility to be included in the study was absence of serious cognitive impairment. The interviewers were three psychiatrists who were trained in the use of the interview schedule by the principal investigator. One of the interviewers had participated in a previous qualitative study (Cross-cultural applicability research study on alcohol and drugs). The present study was conducted in different settings for reasons of convenience. Professionals and policy-makers were interviewed at their places of work, while patients were interviewed at home or at the place where they were cared for. Family members were interviewed at home or workplace. Participants were explained the purpose of the study, and were asked to sign consent form. The interviewer kept detailed notes of each interview. After the interview, participants completed the self-administered questionnaires.

Pile-sorting and concept mapping

Pile sorting and concept mapping were carried out from March to May 1997. Participants were selected through a procedure similar to that followed for the key informant interviews study. Professionals were notified beforehand of the exercise by the principal investigator and patients and family members by the principal investigator and their physician. An interview was arranged with the participant by the interviewer, at the individual's convenience: it was carried out in the workplace, at home, or at the study headquarters. At the start, participants were given a brief description of the study and its purpose, and the tasks they had to perform. A set of 90 cards in Greek, as requested, was then presented to the participant, together with blank cards for naming piles with a request to form piles. No time limit was set, but no participant exceeded 70 minutes. The interviewer then wrote the numbers of the cards and the names and reasons for piles on prepared forms.

After that exercise was finished, participants were given the study questionnaire and asked to complete it in accordance with the written instructions provided. The questionnaire and written instructions were presented in Greek translation. The instructions included the basic descriptions of impairment, activity and participation, as defined in ICIDH-2, and guidelines for completing the schedule. Participants were asked to complete the questionnaires within 15 days. With a few exceptions, most of them completed the procedure in the required time. Help with the structure and the rules for completing the questionnaire was provided by the interviewer, either at the time of presenting the schedule to the participant, or when it was returned if the respondent had any queries. In this case, some extra time was given to him/her to complete it fully.

Results

Linguistic analysis

Four types of problems were identified and described during the linguistic analysis from English into Greek and the back-translation of the terms.

A few terms were found to be difficult to translate into the Greek language, because no equivalent terms exist in Greek, or the term acquires a different meaning when translated. Back-translation (if the term is translated) usually results in completely different English terms in these cases. Examples of this kind are the terms "affect" (which can be translated only as a paraphrase, which still does not reflect the exact meaning of the English term), "empathy" (a term correctly back-translated, but with the Greek translation having a completely different meaning from that intended in English), "interference" (meaning mainly hindrance with a negative connotation), and "leisure and civic life."

Secondly, some terms, when translated, either contained only part of the connotation of the original term, or acquired an additional set of connotations, thus changing the meaning of the original. Such terms are "impairment" (which has a general meaning usually not implying health conditions), "disability" (referring in everyday language to incompetence or impotence), "handicap" (usually not referring to health problems), "mobility" and "consciousness."

Thirdly, some of the translated terms overlapped. Examples of such terms overlapping are: disease/disorder/illness/sickness; impairment/disability/disablement; and civic life/community life/social relationships. Each of these translated into a single term in Greek.

Fourthly, some English terms were modified both in the translation and in the examples provided. Such terms include "consciousness," "empathy," "affect," "civic and community life."

Key informant interviews and self-administered questionnaires

Qualitative analysis

The analysis of the interviews produced some interesting results. First, in Section A, none of the key informants used the term "impaired" or "handicapped" to define the conditions described. Instead, most of the participants spoke of disabled persons or of persons with disability. The same terms were used in the other two questions (though not by the majority in the third question, referring to social participation/handicap), indicating that disability and disablement are used as general terms to define the consequences of diseases.

In general, thresholds for noticing, seriousness and needing help, for all five of the conditions explored, agreed with those obtained in the other cultures involved in the study. Hence, thresholds for noticing a mobility problem include the visible signs of the problem, but also, in Greece, signs of irritability and nervousness. For mental disorders, thresholds include, among the other signs mentioned by most sites in the study, dangerousness. Notably, aggressive behaviour was also mentioned, in common with a few other cultures, with regard to heroin problems.

In the area of social participation and obtaining employment, participants felt that people would be most surprised if a psychotic person or a person with a heroin problem kept a full-time job, and that such persons would be more likely to face barriers than those using wheelchairs. There is a general trend towards higher stigma for mental disorders, compared with physical disabilities. Individuals with physical disabilities were described by informants as occasioning less surprise concerning their integration in work, and they were thought to be much less likely to face barriers of a social nature. The prospect of getting married and having a family was viewed much less favourably for persons with mental health problems, but especially with alcohol and substance abuse or low intelligence. In general, among all five conditions, attitudes were much less favourable to mental health patients, followed by persons with low intelligence, heroin addicts and persons with alcohol problems. The most favourable attitudes were recorded for people with mobility problems.

It was generally recognized by the key informants that assistance is needed for persons suffering from these problems, although it was generally felt that assistance for persons with alcohol or drug problems should include only treatment and practical assistance, and not financial support. It was also suggested that all support for this group should be time-limited and contingent on progress towards overcoming the addiction.

The key informants discussed differing etiology for several conditions, and the impact that this would have on public support for the provision of services or both mobility and mental health problems, it was felt that a problem resulting after a car accident would attract more sympathy than self-inflicted problems. For alcohol and drug problems, starting after a psychosocial problem such as the death of a family member would also attract more sympathy and tolerance, although in these cases the support would be time-limited.

Quantitative analysis

Social disapproval/stigma ratings

Of the 18 different conditions included in the investigation, the least stigmatizing were being obese, blind or unable to read. The three most stigmatizing were being HIV-positive, having a drug addiction, and having a criminal record for burglary.

Public reaction ratings

The three conditions that were rated as attracting the least negative reactions in Greece were a woman being in the eight month of pregnancy, being blind, and being obese. The three conditions attracting the most negative reactions for people appearing in public were being under the influence of drugs, being visibly drunk, and having chronic active psychosis.

Rank-order of disabilities

According to the results of the rank-order exercise, the three most disabling conditions were regarded as being quadriplegia, active psychosis and dementia. The disabilities that ranked as the least disabling were vitiligo on the face, infertility, and rheumatoid arthritis.

Activities

The average likelihood that people would be surprised if the person did the listed activity was calculated for all five health conditions and each of the 10 activities. The results ranked the conditions in the following order, from highest to lowest, of likelihood that they would elicit surprise: low intelligence, active psychosis, heroin problem, alcohol problem and mobility problem. The same procedure was repeated for the likelihood of facing restrictions or barriers in performing these activities. The results were similar, with the one difference that active psychosis was first, followed by low intelligence. These two disabilities appear to be judged as having the most impact on the person's ability to engage in the activities, and to meet the expectations of the public.

Pile sorting

The number of piles ranged from 6 to 27, with a mean number of 12. By use of the QAP statistical procedure in ANTHROPAC, Greek data showed a correlation of 0.854 with the overall data (all sites combined), indicating a high level of correspondence with the consensus structure for the relationships among the items that make up the classification. The visual results of Johnson's hierarchical cluster analysis show 10 clusters of items, very similar to those obtained by analyzing the overall data. However, some differences can be observed: for example the number of items in the Greek clusters varied from 2 to 15, while in the overall data it ranged from 5 to 13.

Concept mapping

For all 90 items in the common list for the concept mapping study, we calculated the percentage of people who had problems with the item in the first eight questions of the questionnaire. Only a few items were regarded as prob-

Table 1. Problematic items and dimensions: Results from the concept mapping in Greece

Clarification needed
Interacting with an equal/co-worker/peer (item)
Keeping appropriate physical contact, and maintenance of social space (item)
Communication content (item)

Culturally sensitive (taboo)
Transferring oneself
Keeping appropriate physical contact, and maintenance of social space
Dating and forming a sexual relationship
Handling body – attached technical aids
Sexual functions
Performing consensual sexual acts
Responding to dangers

lematic, following the rule of considering them to be so if more than 25% of the subjects expressed such a view. Table 1 contains these items.

The results presented in Table 1 indicate that most items function quite well within the Greek cultural context, with a few notable exceptions. Items related to interaction, either at work or involving physical contact, are not easily understood in Greek society. All items related to sexual relationships were regarded as sensitive. Surprisingly items related to movement (transferring oneself), technical aids and response to dangers were also regarded as culturally sensitive.

With regards to the distinction between the concepts of impairments, activity and participation, it is worth noting that only in 15 of the 90 items did

Table 2. Ranking of most important items in Greece according to the concept mapping procedure *(% of rating 4)*

1. Thought, abstraction, judgement and related executive functions (82%)
2. Transferring oneself (76%)
3. Memory (76%)
4. Motor coordination (76%)
5. Visual sensory functions (72%)
6. Orientation (72%)
7. Seeing (69%)
8. Taking care of one's health (69%)
9. Selfcare (69%)
10. Intellectual development and function (69%)
11. Consciousness (69%)
12. Moving around (69%)
13. Using public transport (69%)

more than 75% of the respondents place items in the appropriate category according to ICIDH-2 Beta-1 draft. In 47 items, more than half of the respondents placed them at the appropriate category. This indicates that the basic structure and concepts of the ICIDH-2 are not widely known, so that considerable effort must be devoted to training and education to ensure their appropriate application.

Thirteen items, included in Table 2, were considered the most important. These are. Taking care of pets, dressing, and cooking, baking and frying solids were considered to be the least important items.

Conclusion

The findings of the cultural study lead to certain conclusions, which are similar in most instances to those obtained in other cultures participating in this project. The majority of the items in ICIDH-2 are important for the application of ICIDH-2 as a global frame of reference and a common language for the description, recording and assessment of disability. These are important for our country, so that this frame of reference can be applied in the future in the different fields related to disability. It is clear that to achieve a culturally sensitive translation of ICIDH-2 and the assessment instruments and procedures related to it, the cultural issues outlined above need to be taken into account.

The Greek language is rich and elaborate, and such a translation is possible. However, the annotations and examples must be changed in the case of terms not easily applied to the culture. The terms themselves have to be translated taking into account that the concepts underlying the terms have to be implied by reference to them. A further point relating to the basic concepts of the ICIDH-2, which is evident from both the key informant interviews and the concept mapping studies, is the lack of familiarity with the concepts of impairment, disability/activity limitation and handicap/participation restriction. This is explained by the fact that the previous version of the classification was not widely accepted and used.

As in most sites taking part in this project, the findings of the key informant interview study indicate the lack of parity between physical and mental disability. Public opinion attach greater stigma to mental health conditions, including those relating to drugs and alcohol and to mental subnormality. Physical disability attract more sympathy, more opportunities are provided for them, and they prompt less public reaction.

The rank-ordering of health conditions showed, as expected, that the most chronic and incurable diseases are considered more disabling. Among them, mental disorders such as chronic psychosis and dementia are considered to be very disabling. On the other hand, treatable conditions are considered less disabling.

An interesting finding from the pile sorting study is that people in Greece and in all the other countries participating in the study share similar views and perceptions as regards the descriptions of disability and the relationships between concepts. This indicates that a universally applicable classification that is also culturally sensitive is possible.

Chapter 7
India – Bangalore

R. Srinivasa Murthy, S. Chatterji, C.R. Chandrasekhar, and K. Sekar [*]

Highlights from CAR study in Bangalore, India

- In southern India, and particularly in Bangalore, services for persons with disability associated with physical and mental disorders are far more developed than in the rest of the country.

- Though terms such as impairment, disability and handicap do not exist in Kannada, with a few exceptions most terms in ICIDH-2 could be conceptually translated into the language.

- Awareness regarding the law, facilities and programmes and utilization of available benefits is limited.

- Stigma associated with mental disorders and related disability is high and has a greater role producing "handicap" than the actual disability experienced by persons with these disorders.

- Disability associated with mental disorders is recognized as a dynamic and changing phenomenon as compared to that associated with physical disorders.

- Alcohol and drug-related disorders were the most stigmatized and elicited the strongest public reaction.

- Mental health conditions were ranked in the middle range amongst disabling conditions.

- Most respondents's conceptual map of the area of disability closely resembles the framework of ICIDH-2

- There is a clear need to increase awareness and improve services with regard to persons with disability due to both physical and mental disorders.

[*] National Institute of Mental Health and Neurosciences, Bangalore, Karnataka, India.

Introduction

The city of Bangalore is located in the southern part of India; its population is 5 million. The city is the capital of Karnataka state which is one of the country's 30 states. The estimated current population of India is 996 million. The city and state of Karnataka are covered by all the Indian laws and programmes. The city is the fifth largest city in India. Its special characteristics are its high growth rate in the last 30 years, the presence of advanced information technology centres (more than 250 software companies) and the cosmopolitan nature of the population. The city is also home to the National Institute of Mental Health and Neuro Sciences, which is a premier institution for mental health and neurosciences. This institution is a postgraduate training centre, with a 850-bed hospital, and a major centre for research. It carried out the CAR study in this part of India. Other characteristics of the city are a high literacy rate, a large industrial worker population and very high vehicular density. The state of Karnataka is one of the top five states in the country for both health indices and general development.

Bangalore is home to a large number of institutional and community-based facilities for persons with disabilities, far in excess of the national average. Many governmental and nongovernmental agencies are engaged in working with the disabled in the city.

Some years ago, the Indian Parliament adopted the *Persons with Disabilities Act, 1996*, which has changed the status of disabled individuals. Prior to this Act, the efforts to improve the quality of life of persons with disability were largely confined to the voluntary sector. The new Act has a wide variety of provisions to promote full participation, protection of rights and equal opportunities. An important aspect of the Act is the statutory requirement to set up administrative structures at the national and state levels. There is also a requirement that representatives of disabled persons be members of the various committees. Mental illness is recognized as being linked to disabilities and this is the first step towards removing discrimination. Since the formulation of the Act, there has been a quantum leap in activities for disabled individuals. To name two of them, the Ministry of Welfare and Social Justice has formulated schemes in order to support disability-related activities, while the Ministry of Rural Development through its CAPART Division, has provided support to over 50 organizations for community-based rehabilitation in rural areas. These are in addition to the funding support provided from international organizations such as Action Aid. The mass media are also sensitive to the needs and rights of disabled persons and there has recently been an increased coverage of disability-related issues in the print and audio-visual media.

To support these emerging national developments, there are national institutes for mental retardation (Secunderabad), the hearing handicapped (Mumbai), the orthopaedically handicapped (Calcutta), the visually handicapped (Dehradun) and mental health and neurosciences (Bangalore).

One of the most striking aspects of the disability field in India is the vast regional differences across the country. In general, southern India has more facilities than northern or north-eastern parts of the country.

The national level organizations such as the National Association for the Blind and the Federation for the Welfare of the Mentally Handicapped are playing a vital role in the emerging disability programmes and policies with their proactive involvement.

Methods

Components of the study

Linguistic analysis

The methodology involved translation and back-translation of the draft version of the ICDIH-2. The translation was conceptual rather than verbatim or literal. The translation process sought the closest cultural equivalent. The evaluation exercise included:

* Identification of problems
* Synonyms in local language
* Avoiding jargon
* Gender and age applicability
* Back translation

Focus group study

In total five focus groups were conducted at the Bangalore centre. The groups consisted of:

* Individuals with disability related to mental illness (one group)
* Family members/care-givers of disabled persons (one group)
* Health care professionals (three groups)

The themes selected for the focus groups were:

1. General disability model
2. Parity, stigmatization and social participation
3. Current practices and needs

All the above three themes were used in the three professional focus groups. The care-givers/family members discussed themes 2 and 3 (stigmatization and social participation and current practices and needs). Group 1, consisting of persons with disability related to mental disorders, discussed theme 3 (current practices and needs).

The participants in the focus groups consisting of professionals were working in the field of alcohol, drug, mental illness, orthopaedic, visual and other handicaps. Both medical and non-medical personnel were involved. These professionals were sent an initial letter by post informing them of the purpose and procedures of the study and inviting them to take part in a focus group. Once their willingness to participate had been obtained, they were given confirmation of the date, time and venue by telephone. All members were paid Rs. 250 to cover their incidental costs.

The care-givers/family members and persons with disability related to mental disorders were selected from the inpatient psychiatry wards of NIMHANS in Bangalore. These individuals were selected a day or two prior to the focus group meeting. They were informed about the procedure by the field investigators. When they expressed willingness to participate and their current clinical condition had been assessed, and after informed consent had been obtained, two groups of care-givers and persons with disability related to mental disorders were formed.

Two professionals conducted the focus groups. The senior faculty member (CRC) moderated the groups and the research investigator made a process record of the interviews. All of the focus groups were video- and audiotaped for compilation of the final report. Except for one focus group, which considered the general disability model, all other focus groups were conducted in Kannada.

Key informant interview and self-administered questions

Seventeen subjects participated in the key informant interviews and 16 of them completed the self-administered questionnaire. The sample consisted of three medical professionals, three alcohol and drug abuse health care-givers, three physically disabled persons, three specialists and three policy-makers. Of the key informants, six were women and eleven were men.

The respondents were chosen using a focused convenience sampling procedure. Potential subjects were written a letter or contacted over the telephone;

the purpose and nature of the study were then explained. The alcohol and drug abuse and physically disabled subjects were recruited in the same manner. Two trained psychologists conducted the key informant interviews and the self-administered questionnaire component. Prior to the interview, respondents signed an informed consent form and completed a face sheet giving demographic details. The interviewer briefly described the purpose of the study and proceeded with the interview. These interviews were not tape-recorded and the interviewer wrote down all the answers. Following the interview the subjects completed the rank-order task. The self-administered questionnaires were left with the respondents, who were requested to complete and return them.

Concept mapping and pile sort

Pile sorting is a systematic technique which allows the participants to create a culturally appropriate classification of the cultural domain. The pile sort list consisted of 90 items. The respondent made piles of the terms, based on perceived similarities or differences. On completion of each set of the piles they were asked to label them.

A sample of 30 completed the concept mapping and 26 of them completed the pile sorting instruments. Three of the 30 subjects completed the Kannada version of the instruments. Two people were not educated, and so were not able to complete the pile sort. The procedure to obtain the samples was the same as for the key informant interviews, except for a few respondents for concept mapping who were recruited from a community health clinic.

The Bangalore centre chose an additional 10 concepts to be included in the concept mapping matrix. They were: acting independently in social participation; avoidance behaviour; balancing privacy and socialization; handling own social positions; handling social responsibilities; taking decisions; use of banking or other services to assist in management of money; making adjustments/corrections to planned sequence of activities; intimate relationships; and acquiring new skills.

For the concept mapping and pile sorting components each subject signed the consent form and completed the face sheet. The researcher briefly described both instruments, provided instructions and left the subjects alone to complete the tasks. The pile sort instrument was completed first, followed by the concept mapping matrix.

Results

Linguistic analysis

The exercise revealed a number of linguistic incompatibilities. The problem terms identified at the Bangalore centre are presented in Table 1:

Table 1. Problematic items identified in linguistic analysis, Bangalore

Original concepts	Problems in translation
Disease, ill, sickness	Synonymous
Structure	Has different meaning
Quality of life, subjective well-being, standard of living	Overlapping
Abstraction and judgement	No equivalent
Non-verbal	Difficult concept
Orientation	No word in Kannada
Use of humour	Difficult to translate

The statements identified as problematic for translation at the Bangalore centre were as follows:

- Appropriate physical contact
- Visual sensory function
- Use of communication devices
- Cooking, baking and frying
- Dating and sexual relations

The concepts of "integrity" and "abstraction" yielded partially equivalent terms/words in Kannada. Similarly, the four words "affect," "disorder," "integrity," and "non-verbal" gave either a poor translation or multiple meanings when translated.

The above-mentioned concepts, phrases and items emerged during translation and back-translation. The words were either interchangable or identically used for two different concepts in the original English.

The translation/back-translation exercise showed that the tool developed and designed in the English language had its own unique characteristics. When it was translated into Kannada, the translator faced many difficulties. There were no equivalent phrases for "disease, illness, sickness," or "quality of life, subjective well-being, standard of living" that could distinguish these individual words and their nuances within the phrases. Difficulties in translating words like impairment, handicap, disability, integrity, abstraction, empathy and affect were also identified. Finally, the problem of choosing between equivalent words and phrases or concepts posed a challenge for the group in arriving at the nearest equivalent terms that are understood by the general public.

Focus group study

The results obtained from the focus groups were as follows:

- It is difficult to translate impairment, disability and handicap into Kannada. Impairment has an equivalent word *"durbalathe."* Disability is translated as *"durbalathe," "ashaktate," "asamarthathe."* Handicap translates as *"addi," "anga-vikalatthe"* meaning obstacle, organ deficit or damaged organ. It is difficult to convey the differences between these three words. *"Durbalathe," "ashaktate"* and *"asamarthathe"* are also popularly used to mean "weakness."

- In India, mental illness is equated with madness. Only severe mental disorders are recognized as "mental illnesses." The general public is not aware of the modern explanations regarding causes of mental illnesses. Nor is it aware of different types of psychoses. *"hutchu," "buddibhramane," "tale kettide"* ("madness," "disturbance of higher mental function," "head has become bad") are the popular terms used to describe "schizophrenia," "mania" and "dementia." Thus the question relating to differences in attitudes to different kinds of "mental disablements" was difficult for respondents from the general population, as they could not see shades of disability in different mental health conditions.

- The mental health services available in India are very meagre. All the existing mental health personnel (2–3 million) are located in big cities. None are available in the rural areas where 755 million people live. Similarly, there are only a few laws related to mental disorders and substance abuse, and they are not known to people.

- The participants had difficulty in understanding and answering the question relating to which "mental disorder related disablements" elicited the most negative response from society. Similarly, the awareness of programmes and the eligibility criteria for these programmes and services was extremely limited.

- In most part of India there is a need to start the services from scratch; hence respondents found it very difficult to respond to the question related to the gap between needs and services.

- People find it easy to accept and understand the concepts of impairment and disability with regard to physical conditions such as blindness, deafness, loss of limb. However, they find it difficult to apply the same concepts to mental disorders and substance abuse. To some extent they understand these constructs with regard to mental retardation, more specifically when it is associated with physical impairment.

Except for excitement and gross negligence of personal care, symptoms of mental disorders do not elicit "negative responses." Other people show severe negative and hostile responses once a person is labelled as "mad." Thus social stigma appears to cause more "handicap" than the illness itself.

Impairment and disability are static and do not change in most cases of disabilities associated with physical health conditions. But in the case of mental disorders and substance abuse, impairment and disability may keep changing. When there is worsening of symptoms such as aggression and neglect of personal hygiene, the disability and handicap increase. Later they may decrease once the acute disturbance has subsided. There should be a provision in the assessment tools to accommodate these changes.

Key informant interview and self-administered questions

Reactions to activities and barriers

Among the five health conditions and performance of the 10 activities taken together, a majority of respondents expressed surprise about a person with a heroin problem being able to carry out the activities. The smallest proportion of respondents were surprised if a person born with low intelligence undertook the activities, followed by a person who hears voices, a person in a wheelchair, and a person with alcohol problems. For the question "Is it likely that anyone would place restriction or barriers?" among the five health conditions, a majority of the respondents felt that "persons who hear voices" face the most barriers and "persons in wheelchair" face the fewest barriers. The intermediate groups were persons born with low intelligence, persons with alcohol problems and persons with a heroin problem, in that order.

Stigma ratings

Of the 18 health conditions presented, the three least stigmatizing conditions were being wheelchair-bound, blindness and inability to read. The three most stigmatizing conditions were HIV positive, criminal record for burglary, and drug addiction.

Public reaction ratings

Of the 10 conditions presented, the three that elicited the most negative reactions were "being under the influence of drugs," "being visibly drunk" and "someone who is dirty and unkempt." The least negative reactions elicited were towards "a woman in her 8th month of pregnancy," "a person who is intellectually slow" and "an obese person."

Rank order of disability

The three conditions perceived to as most disabling were quadriplegia, total blindness and dementia. The three least disabling conditions were infertility, vitiligo on the face, and severe migraine.

Qualitative data summary

The experience of carrying out the key informant interviews showed that it is very difficult in the local culture to get the informants to talk on behalf of the society or the people around them. By and large the respondents relied more on their personal experiences than on being a part of and representing the wider society. There are no general activities that involve all communities in society, and as the society itself is segregated in terms of religion, upper, middle and lower socioeconomic situations and caste groups, the informants found it difficult to report on the society as a whole. In spite of such limitations, specific and marked differences are visible with regard to the five scenarios. Inter- and intra-group variations, assertions, authority and, at times, ambivalence too were seen in the responses. Urban/rural differences, gender differences and differences in economic status were marked in the key informant interviews.

Concept mapping and pile sort

The results for the Bangalore centre revealed 13 clusters. They were: civic and leisure activities; social functioning; sexual functioning; work and economic activities; self-care and daily routine; motor coordination; communication; learning and problem-solving; sensory functions; cognitive functions; psychomotor activity; emergency situations; and psychological functions.

Conclusion

Throughout known history, India has taken a positive attitude to persons with disabilities. There are records of special centres for care of persons with disabilities. There is a high tolerance of all "deviant" behaviour with relatively low stigma unless an individual is a "socially disturbing person." In the whole country, only 20,000 persons (less than 1% of the expected chronically ill persons) with mental impairments are in specialised institutions. All the others are living in the community with their families. On the other hand, Government assistance for persons with disabilities is extremely limited; less than 1% of persons with disabilities receive any meaningful services. The *Persons with Disabilities Act, 1996* has focuses attention on the needs of persons with different disabilities. People's awareness of this progressive Act, however, is limited.

The 1996 Act recognizes categories and degrees of disability. The mentally ill and those with cured leprosy are included along with the visually impaired, hearing impaired, and physically disabled. A person with at least 40% disability is recognized as disabled, and there are also provisions for the severely disabled. An investigator noted that "the measurement and assessment of disability is not uniform and varies greatly from place to place. In the rural areas, there is hardly any standard measurement used."

The CAR study has helped to raise important issues in urban Karnataka and has given the investigators a clearer understanding of the concepts and classifications in the ICIDH-2 and its applicability to the situation in southern India.

Chapter 8
India – Chennai

*R. Thara and T.N. Srinivasan**

Highlights from the CAR study in Chennai (Madras), India

- The concepts and terms used in ICIDH-2, with a few exceptions, were not difficult to convey in the local language, Tamil.
- Excluding alcohol and drug problems, respondents thought that those with mental problems should be treated on a par with those with physical problems, as they have as much disability.
- Patients with mental illness, alcohol problems, and other substance use problems are very much stigmatized and avoided by the public. The law is often against the interests of the mentally ill.
- Stigma and misconceptions about mental illness are widespread and should be removed.
- Many in India are not aware of the recent *Persons with Disabilities Act, 1996* and its provision for the mentally disabled. The Act should be further implemented.
- The mentally disabled and their care-givers should play a dynamic and direct role in fighting for their needs and rights.

Introduction

This report is based on data gathered from the Chennai study site in India. Chennai (formerly known as Madra) is the largest metropolitan city in southern India, with a population of nearly 6 million. It is the administrative capital of

---

* Director and Consultant Psychiatrist, Schizophrenia Research Foundation (India), Chennai, India.

the state of Tamil Nadu. This state, with a population of 60 million, is one of the leading states in the country in the development of the health care system. The main language spoken in the region is Tamil.

The disability situation in India, applicable to Chennai too, is as follows. There is no parity between physical and mental health conditions with respect to equal treatment, benefits, law and public opinion. It was only in 1996 that a parliamentary act (the *Persons with Disabilities Act*) was enacted, placing the mentally ill on a par with the physically disabled. However, this legislation has yet to take effect in practice. There are very few welfare agencies, political backers, self-help groups, advocacy groups, or employment and educational opportunities for the mentally disabled. The physically disabled are treated comparatively better in these respects, but the facilities available are still not enough to meet their needs.

Methods

Components of the study

There were five components of the Chennai CAR study:
1. Translation and linguistic analysis;
2. Concept mapping;
3. Pile sorting;
4. Key informant interview; and
5. Focus group study.

Translation and linguistic analysis

At the Chennai centre, terms and concepts in the Tamil language were compared with those in English. The standard translation/back-translation procedure was adopted.

Concept mapping

Concept mapping was carried out to determine the content and limits of disability domains. The respondents were asked to respond to a matrix of 10 questions for each of 90 items (disability concepts) and encouraged to comment on the applicability and relevance of each of the items.

Pile sorting

Pile sorting was done to define and analyse assessment domains from a cluster of 90 items. These items were selected from the draft ICIDH-2, representing all impairments and major domains related to activity and participation. The respondents were asked to sort the items into groups based on similarities and differences.

Key informant interview

The key informant interview is a culturally sensitive method that allows the application of statistical tools to produce hierarchical and relational schemes of disabilities across cultures and professions. The interview was conducted in two parts, requiring the completion of two schedules, The key informant interview schedule (consisting of four sections – terms and concepts, thresholds and causes, ranking of disability, and degree of social disapproval and public reaction to the disabled) and the self-administered key informant questionnaire. The analysis also looked at variations in the opinions expressed on physical and mental disabilities.

Focus group study

The focus groups were conducted with the objective of exploring (a) the stigma attached to disabilities in the culture and (b) current practices and needs related to disabilities in the society. A total of five focus groups, with eight to 10 individuals in each, were conducted.

The respondents

Thirty subjects were recruited to carry out the concept mapping and pile sorting exercise. This group consisted of 15 professionals working in the area of physical and/or mental disability and 15 persons affected with a disability or their care-givers. For the key informant interview, 15 subjects who did not participate in the concept mapping-pile sorting exercise were involved. They included three persons each from among professionals in the mental health field, physical disability experts, persons with mental disability or their care-givers, persons with physical disability or their care-givers and policy-makers in the disability field. The five focus groups were made up of individuals with mental and physical disabilities, care-givers of mentally and physically disabled people, and health and social service professionals working in the disability field. All respondents were residents of the urban area of the city of Madras. Only those who gave their consent to participate in the study were included. Confidentiality of identity was guaranteed.

Results

Translation and linguistic analysis

There were very few terms that were difficult to translate into Tamil (e.g., "abstraction," "judgement," "executive functions," "consciousness"). Such items were more clearly conveyed by explanatory phrases. The most frequent problem was overlap in the meaning of the concepts used in the local language (e.g., disease and disorder, impairment and illness, disability and disablement, quality of life and standard of living).

Concept mapping

Difficulty in understanding the terms and their definitions was expressed by only a minority of the respondents (ranging from 10% to 20%). All the items were scored at a middle level on the scale of importance for inclusion in ICIDH-2. The problematic items from the concept mapping are listed in Table 1.

Table 1. Concept mapping: problematic items in Chennai

Type of difficulty	ICIDH-2 item
Applicable in culture	Dating and forming relationships Sexual functions
Use for all ages	Planning and organizing meals Taking care of meals Dating and forming relationships Sexual functions Performing consensual sexual acts
Use for both genders	Cooking, baking, frying solids Dating and forming relationships
Use for all social/economic groups	Dating and forming relationships
Use for all ethnic/minority groups	Dating and forming relationships
Cultural taboo	Dating and forming relationships Sexual functions Performing consensual sexual acts

Pile sorting

The respondents from Madras grouped the 90 items into 14 piles. They were: civic and leisure activities, social functioning, sexual functioning, work and economic activities, self-care and daily routine, motor coordination, communication, learning and problem solving, sensory functions, cognitive functions, psychomotor activity, emergency situations, psychological functions, organizing and monitoring. The largest numbers of items were placed in the clusters on self-care and daily routine, motor coordination, and communication.

Key informant interview and self-administered questionnaire

Qualitative analysis (terms and concepts, thresholds and causes)

Analysis of the key informant interviews revealed that the informants were not able to differentiate the different constructs of impairment, disability and handicap. There were no equivalent terms in the local language that could demarcate the three concepts. The meaning of the concepts was clearly understood, but they were collectively termed in Tamil the equivalent of the English "handicap." The informants were not able to differentiate mild and severe forms of disabilities.

In comparing physical and mental disability, the informants felt that marriage and getting a job would be difficult for both categories, though more so for the mentally disabled. Those with alcohol and drug problem were perceived as more easily being able to find a job or get married, but were thought to have more difficulty in doing well in both responsibilities. Group members were unanimous in saying that the physically and mentally disabled should receive assistance from the Government, though they were not sure about the duration of disability for deciding on eligibility. They were unanimous again in saying that alcohol and drug abusers did not deserve any aid from the Government. Thus, the informants expressed the need for parity between physical disability, and mental disability but not for substance dependence.

Disability caused at birth or due to an accident or bereavement drew more sympathy and understanding though this was limited to physical and mental disability only, not alcohol and drug dependence.

Quantitative analysis

Rank-order of disability
The three conditions perceived to cause maximum disability were quadriplegia, dementia and total blindness (ranked 1–3 in a ranking order of 1–17). The three disorders felt to be least disabling were severe migraine, vitiligo on the face, and infertility (ranks 15–17). Active psychosis was ranked 5 and major depression 6. Alcoholism and drug addiction were given a lower rankings of 10 and 11, respectively (see Table 2).

Table 2. Comparison of disability rankings: total sample and Chennai site

Health condition (rank in total sample)	Rank in Chennai sample
Quadriplegia (1)	1
Dementia (2)	2
Active psychosis (3)	5
Paraplegia (4)	4
Total blindness (5)	3
Major depression (6)	6
Drug dependence (7)	11
HIV-positivity (8)	7
Alcoholism (9)	10
Total deafness (10)	9
Mild mental retardation (11)	12
Incontinence (12)	8
Below-the-knee amputation (13)	14
Rheumatoid arthritis (14)	13
Severe migraines (15)	15
Infertility (16)	17
Vitiligo on face (17)	16

Note: Ranking ranges from 1 (most disabling) to 17 (least disabling)

Degree of stigma
Of the 18 health conditions presented, the informants responded that the three most stigmatizing conditions were drug addiction, HIV seropositivity, and a criminal record of burglary (a degree of disapproval of 9 on a scale from 0 to 10). The least stigmatizing were using a wheelchair, blindness, and inability to read. Chronic mental disorder drew a disapproval rating of 7, and alcohol problems a rating of 8 on a scale up to 10 (see Table 3).

Table 3. Mean stigma scores for 18 health conditions

Description of the condition	Mean stigma score
Wheelchair-bound	1.6
Borderline intelligence	2.5
Alcoholism	7.8
Drug addiction	8.7
HIV-positivity	9.1
Homeless	3.3
Criminal record	8.7
Depression	3.1
Blindness	1.9
Leprosy	6.3
Chronic mental disorder	6.7
Being dirty and unkempt	7.2
Inability to read	1.9
Dementia	4.1
Obese	3.0
Does not take care of children	5.8
Facial disfigurement	3.7
Cannot hold a job	3.1

Note: Stigma rating ranges from 0 (least stigmatized) to 10 (most stigmatized)

Reaction to disabled persons in public

All informants felt that the general public would feel uneasy and tend to avoid a person with alcohol or drug problems, or a dirty and unkempt person. More than two-thirds expressed the same opinion with regard to a mentally ill person. In contrast, informants reported that members of the public would not pay much attention if they saw a woman in an advanced stage of pregnancy or an obese person (see Table 4).

Table 4. Societal reaction to the disabled person in public

Condition of the person appearing in public	Not an issue N (%)		Uneasy/avoid N (%)	
Mental disorder	4	(27)	11	(73)
8th month of pregnancy	14	(93)	1	(7)
In wheelchair	8	(60)	6	(40)
Low intelligence	10	(63)	4	(27)
Dirty and unkempt	1	(7)	14	(93)
Facial disfigurement	5	(23)	10	(67)
Obese	11	(63)	4	(27)
Influence of drug	0	(0)	15	(100)
Influence of alcohol	0	(0)	15	(100)
Blind	7	(47)	7	(47)

Reaction to activities and barriers to them (self-administered questionnaire)
This exercise recorded individuals' possible reactions to a disabled person engaging in different activities normally performed by non-disabled persons, and
informants' views regarding restrictions that might be placed on the disabled
performing the activities. The average ratings for the likelihood that "people
would be surprised if the person did this activity" across all the 10 activities
were calculated for each of the five disability case scenarios. The results revealed that persons with the following disorders would be most likely to elicit
surprise if they engaged in activities similar to the non-disabled: heroin addiction (least surprise); alcohol problems; hearing voices; being wheelchair-bound;
and born with low intelligence (most surprise) (see Table 5).

In the same way, the average ratings for the likelihood that "anyone would
place restrictions or barriers on the person" were calculated. Persons with
the following disabilities were most likely to face barriers: a person who
hears voices (least barrier), with alcohol problems, with heroin addiction, in
a wheelchair, and born with low intelligence (greatest barrier).

Table 5. Performance of activities by type of disability: likelihood of surprise and
likelihood of barriers (in percentage)

Activity	1		2		3		4		5	
	S	R	S	R	S	R	S	R	S	R
Keep home tidy	53	40	13	13	53	20	60	27	60	27
Use public transport	80	60	7	13	33	60	13	27	13	27
In love	27	40	13	40	53	67	47	60	47	60
Sex in relationship	53	40	20	40	33	60	13	33	13	33
Parenting	27	13	40	33	47	53	47	40	47	40
Community activity	27	27	0	7	40	53	40	40	40	40
Manage money	7	20	60	60	33	47	60	67	60	67
Get housing	47	53	47	53	33	60	40	40	40	40
Full-time job	20	27	33	27	53	60	73	53	73	53
Elected to government post	40	33	80	60	67	67	67	67	67	67
Average	38.1	35.3	31.3	34.6	44.5	54.7	46	45.4	52	45.4

Key: S= Surprised; R=Restrictions expected.
Types of disability: 1= confined to wheelchair; 2= low intelligence; 3= psychosis;
          4= alcoholism; 5= drug dependence.

Focus group

The major observations made by the focus groups concerned the lack of
parity between the mentally and the physically disabled, and the scarcity of

facilities and benefits for the disabled. It was noted that existing facilities are mostly in urban settings, with very poor access for most of the disabled in the community. There was thought to be poor awareness of the facilities available for the disabled. The groups felt that the mentally ill were stigmatized because of the misconceptions people have about the causation of these illnesses. They were unhappy that the law was against the interests of the mentally ill. Finally, the focus groups believed that the disabled and their care-givers need to adopt a more dynamic and direct role in fighting for their needs and rights, and not to let the whole burden be borne by the Government as is happening currently. They felt that this was especially true for the mentally disabled. Persons with psychiatric disability made similar comments: "The stigma of schizophrenia will be much lessened if you call me 'chemically imbalanced' and not 'mentally ill'. It gives respect as it sounds equivalent to a chemical problem like diabetes." And: "If I can get a job and earn something, people will look upon me with dignity."

Conclusion

The terms and concepts in ICIDH-2

The respondents in the CAR study did not find the terms and definitions featuring in ICIDH-2 too difficult to comprehend. This suggests that difficulties arising from lack of understanding of the concepts and terms would not be significant in applying ICIDH-2 to describing and measuring disabilities in Chennai. The difficulties in translation into Tamil, which were probably also experienced in other languages, could be overcome by adding descriptive phrases or using terms borrowed from another language that are easily understood by the respondents.

Status of psychiatric disability

Respondents' views that psychiatric disorders cause much disability, are severely stigmatized, and need to be treated on a par with physical disability reconfirm earlier observations (Wig et al. 1980; Prabhu et al. 1984). However, respondents viewed alcohol and drug problems differently. The need felt by people with psychiatric disorders and their family members to reduce the stigma they experience highlights the importance of the issue of stigma in mental illness. In a country where a consumer movement on the part of the mentally disabled is absent, the need for patients and their family members to join together to take up the issue on a major scale was noted by the participants. The groups' observations on the poor state of psychiatric care facilities in the country and their near-total absence in rural areas is again a major issue, as the result is lack of treatment and hence chronic permanent disability.

Overall, it was found that the opinions expressed by lay respondents who were less informed about psychiatric disorders and disability were not significantly different from those elicited from disability experts. Earlier studies have made similar observations (Nunally 1961; Basumallick & Bhattacharya 1983). The CAR study has brought into focus several issues that could help in the development of ICIDH-2 and instruments to measure disabilities that could be applied uniformly in different cultures and countries.

Chapter 9
India – Delhi

*S. Saxena, H. Pal, and U. Singh**

Highlights from CAR study in Delhi, India

- In north India, disability associated with mental and alcohol- and drug-related disorders is much more discriminated against than physical disability.
- There is a general paucity of facilities and services for the disabled in both governmental and nongovernmental sectors. The available services are concentrated in urban areas.
- Awareness regarding the law, facilities and programmes and utilization of available benefits is poor.
- There is a considerable felt need for improvement in the facilities, services and opportunities for disabled people.
- The *Persons with Disabilities Act, 1996*, is a progressive step, but its implementation is very limited.
- The model of disability in ICIDH-2 is acceptable for the scientific community, but a simpler adaptation that can be readily understood should be used for the general public.

Introduction

India is a large country, with an area of 3.1 million km² and a population of nearly 1000 million people. The population density is 301 persons per km². About 73% of the population resides in rural areas and the economy is primarily agrarian. The main language of north India is Hindi. However, many other languages are spoken in the various regions.

* India Institute of Medical Sciences, New Delhi, India.

Health is primarily a concern for the individual states and the administrative structure leaves many decisions regarding particular health issues to the states. The states do not make health a priority issue and in turn depend on central assistance. There are also some central health programmes funded by the central government. The health and social welfare budgets represent a small percentage of the national budget and of GDP. It has been estimated that about 3–5 % of the population has some physical disability, which translates roughly into some 50 million disabled individuals.

Delhi, the centre for the study, is the capital of India and the largest metropolitan city in north India. It has a population of nearly 10 million, a large majority of which is a floating population from nearby towns and states. The population is a mix of various religious, regional and ethnic groups and is truly cosmopolitan in composition. The main language spoken is Hindi.

The present study was carried out to gather information on the understanding of the disablement process and the societal response to it in north India. It was conducted in Delhi, but respondents were selected to roughly represent all segments of society in north India, rather than specifically the city of Delhi. The Delhi centre conducted all the basic components of the CAR study as well as the focus group discussions.

This chapter describes the salient findings of the study and some comparisons with other two sites in south India – Bangalore and Chennai – which are described in Chapters 7 and 8. As similar studies were carried out the methods are not given in detail here.

Results

The results are reported for each individual exercise and then the overall findings are discussed in the concluding section.

Centre description

This information was of a general nature and was offered by the investigators themselves and a few selected consultants who were familiar with the disability situation in north India. It encompassed general cultural views, parity, accommodations made in the society, disability programmes, stigmatization and compensation systems.

The overall state of the disabled was thought to be that of a disadvantaged and neglected segment of society with a high level of stigma and discrimination and a low level of support. Although some steps have been taken recently to enact and implement laws for the benefit of the disabled, overall awareness of them is very poor, partly because of the high illiteracy rate and also because no systematic attempts have been made to educate the public. Governmental facilities and benefits were thought to be meager and largely unavailable to a vast majority.

Opportunities for the disabled are provided by the law, but implementation is unsatisfactory. Out of the allocated 3% of posts reserved for the disabled in certain jobs by the government, less than 1% had been filled according to a recent report. Special education facilities are also not available for the large majority.

Facilities and compensation for disability are organized more systematically for employees of government services (i.e., service civil, the military, and industrial enterprises). Special funds are earmarked for these categories and implementation is more effective. There are also group insurance schemes to provide compensation for disability in service.

Accommodation of the environment for the disabled is at the most basic stage, with a few ramps built in public places. However, there are no signs using Braille or audible signs for hearing impaired people anywhere.

Overall, a degree of social stigma is attached to the disabled. Mental and alcohol/drug-related disabilities are more discriminated against than physical disabilities. However, social tolerance is high, and in the absence of substantial state support, community support – mainly as religious charity – is available. The level of this support differs markedly from region to region and in total it is still far less than required.

Linguistic analysis

This exercise consisted of translation of key terms from English into Hindi, their back-translation and linguistic evaluation following a standard procedure. The key terms were arranged in two lists: list A with 44 items and list B with 67 items. The initial translation was done by experts in disability and the back-translation by a linguistic expert.

Translation procedures employed aimed at conceptual equivalence rather than a literal word-for-word translation. The objective were to:

1. Find the relevant substitute without changing the global meaning (transposition);
2. Operate on notions and not grammatical categories (modulation);
3. Use structural and stylistic means (equivalence);

4. Seek recognizable correspondence between situations (adaptation). The main results of the linguistic analysis are given below.

A total of 17 terms and phrases were identified for evaluation. Overall, however, it was possible to translate the instrument fairly adequately. "Physically intimate" when translated does not convey the import of the original term. Some of the phrases are quite complex and need to be broken into shorter phrases to convey the meaning. For example, "getting along with people" when translated was to read. The phrase "getting around" seems incomplete and lacks specific connotation, which led to an unsatisfactory translation. "Going around one's environment (personal and non-personal)" would convey the meaning more appropriately.

Some of the difficulties in each list and their nature are indicated below.

Linguistic analysis for list A

- "Illness" and "sickness," and "disease" and "disorder" are generally interchangeable.
- "Impairment" is difficult to translate and has no semantic equivalent in Hindi.
- "Handicap" in translation has a meaning closer to deformity than to a disabling condition.
- "Executive function" is difficult to translate.
- "Perception" does not have a good Hindi translation.
- "Use of humour" is not represented in its broad sense by any Hindi term.

Linguistic analysis for list B

Most of the 67 items in list B were easily translatable. Those which were difficult to translate for various reasons are as follows:
- "Transferring" is used to connote movement as in transportation from one location to another rather than personal movement.
- "Keeping appropriate physical contact" runs into cultural barriers as touch has a sexual connotation not present in the original term.
- "Understanding specific signs" is not appropriate, as there is no written language and the illiteracy rate is high.
- "Drinking," by itself, can be understood as drinking alcoholic beverages.
- "Dating" is not a familiar concept.

Key informant interviews

A total sample of 15 individuals was chosen for the key informant interviews. They consisted of three individuals each from among the medical professional category, disability specialists, persons with disability, care-givers, and policy-makers or opinion leaders in the area of disability services.

Social disapproval ratings

The rank-order of the social disapproval ratings of 18 conditions is listed and compared with the All India rating in Table 1. Inability to read met with least and HIV infection met with most disapproval at the Delhi centre. When ratings at all the three Indian centres were combined, the use of drugs was the most disapproved condition, though there was no uniformity in the least disapproved.

Table 1. Rank-order of social disapproval ratings for 18 conditions, Delhi and All India

Item	Delhi	All India
Inability to read	1	1
Obesity	2	3
Depression	3	6
Borderline intelligence	4	5
Blindness	5	4
Demented	6	9
In a wheelchair	7	2
No job	8	10
Homeless	9	7
No child	10	11
Facial disfigurement	11	8
Dirty and ill-kempt	12	12
Using alcohol	13	15
Involved in crime	14	16
Mentally disordered	15	14
Using drugs	16	18
Having leprosy	17	13
Having HIV	18	17

Societal reactions

Societal reactions were assessed in the context of the five scenarios outlined in the protocol; the results are summarized in the tables below. Table 2 records the likelihood that people would express if a person with the particular disability is able to carry out the activity, while Table 3 is about the barriers people with the disability would be expected to face in carrying out the activity.

As far as surprise was concerned, a majority of respondents showed surprise if a person in a wheelchair could keep a job, use public transport, have sex, or hold a government job, and least surprised if the person could manage money matters. For an individual with low intelligence, the most surprise was shown for managing money and least for keeping a job or using public transport in Delhi. At the other centres, however, participation in community functions and using public transport would evoke least surprise, and maximum surprise would be occasioned by holding a government job. For a person who hears voices, keeping things tidy would be most surprising, according to respondents at Delhi as well as other centres, and the least surprising would be use of public transport. For a person with alcohol and drug problem, keeping things tidy and holding a government job would be very surprising at Delhi as well as all centres together and the least surprising would be using public transport and having sex.

As far as societal barriers were concerned, sex was thought most difficult for an individual in a wheelchair, and people would place fewest barriers in the way of a person with mental retardation keeping things tidy. Barriers were likely to be placed also in the way of persons with mental retardation or with drug and alcohol use problems holding a government job.

Table 2. Surprise if people with disabilities carry out specified activities, Delhi and All India (% surprised)

Activity	S1		S2		S3		S4		S5	
	Delhi	All India	Delhi	All India	Delhi	All India	Delhi	All India	Delhi	All India
Keep things tidy	73	66	20	17	68	59	80	72	73	62
Use public transport	86	84	20	13	27	30	20	15	20	18
Love	66	43	53	28	53	52	27	35	33	37
Have sex	86	60	43	24	50	44	20	13	27	22
Parenting	53	37	57	40	68	50	47	46	43	43
Community activity	33	30	27	13	33	37	47	35	57	43
Manage money	20	8	80	63	53	44	33	48	60	58
Find apartment	33	39	67	52	53	46	20	33	47	45
Job hold	46	34	67	44	67	53	47	59	80	76
Government job	73	52	73	76	80	70	60	61	87	79

Table 3. Likelihood of facing barriers in undertaking activities, Delhi and All India (% somewhat/very likely)

Activity	S1		S2		S3		S4		S5	
	Delhi	All India	Delhi	All India	Delhi	All India	Delhi	All India	Delhi	All India
Keep things tidy	33	43	7	7	33	26	40	33	27	24
Use public transport	40	60	20	22	60	48	27	26	27	26
Love	60	54	73	52	67	65	67	59	73	61
Have sex	80	60	64	49	71	60	53	39	57	41
Parenting	26	26	43	33	47	50	47	39	50	43
Community activity	20	23	33	17	53	54	60	46	57	46
Manage money	26.7	21	60	67	53	48	40	50	73	66
Find apartment	53	50	60	61	60	57	33	37	47	47
Job hold	26	28	47	33	60	57	60	50	60	53
Government job	40	34	73	70	73	72	53	67	73	67

Key: S1 = person in wheelchair; S2 = person born with low intelligence; S3 = person who hears voices; S4 = person with alcohol problems; S5 = person with heroin problem.

Public reactions

Public reactions to various disabilities were assessed. It was found that they were most extreme for facial disfigurement and the use of drugs and alcohol. Table 4 gives details.

Table 4. Reactions to appearance in public of individuals with various health conditions, Delhi and All India (% strong reactions and rank)

Item	Delhi		All India	
	%	Rank	%	Rank
Facial disfigurement	80	1	74	1
Publicly drunk	33	2	46	3
Mental disorders	13	3	17	4
Obesity	7	4	7	6
Blindness	7	4	7	6
Eight month of pregnancy	7	4	4	7
Using drugs	–	–	67	2
Dirty/unkempt	0		17	4
Intellectually slow	0		4	7

Concept mapping and pile sorting

Concept mapping and pile sorting techniques were used to identify the cultural properties of items and their interrelationship in hierarchical and relational schemes. A list of 90 items was selected from the ICIDH-2 draft and presented as cards. Respondents were asked to classify the items into separate categories on the basis of similarities and differences and to state the reasons for their categorization.

A total of 30 individuals completed the exercise at the Delhi centre. They consisted of 15 members each from the medical health professional category and the care-givers category. The latter category included 5 individuals concerned with physical disability and 10 with ADM-related disability. Items that more than 25% of participants found problematic for various domains are set out in Table 5.

Table 5. Problematic items for more than 25% of participants

Type of problem	Item	
Usability in all age groups	14	Keeping appropriate distance
	17	Economic self-sufficiency
	37	Citizenship responsibilities
	51	Planning and organizing
	67	Cooking, baking, frying
	71	Dating and forming
	77	Sexual function
	83	Performing consensual sex
Usability for both genders	51	Planning and organizing
	67	Cooking, baking, frying
	71	Dating and forming relationships
Usability in culture	71	Dating and forming relationships
	77	Sexual function
	83	Performing consensual sex
Use in all socioeconomic groups	71	Dating and forming relationships
Ethnic/minority	71	Dating and forming relationships
Cultural Sensitivity	71	Dating and forming relationships
	77	Sexual function
	83	Performing consensual sex

Focus groups

For the focus groups a logically laid predetermined interview guide containing questions for discussion was used. The themes were "Parity, stigmatization and social participation" which referred to the exploration of the stigma attached to disability in the culture, and "Current practices and needs," which referred to current practices and the needs of people with and care-givers of people with disability.

Two researchers, one of whom was the coordinator and the other the rapporteur, conducted all the groups. Verbatim quotes were recorded whenever needed to give detail and explain participants' views. The descriptive analysis discussed the findings of the focus groups by summarizing and providing the clearest possible understanding of the issues. Relational analysis focused on the range and depth of variation, highlighting differences between sexes, experts and lay persons and differences in social or economic groups.

All groups were homogeneous in constitution Five group discussions were held at the Delhi Centre. Two groups focused on the "Current practices and needs," one consisting of individuals with physical disability (10 members) and the other of health professionals (10 members). Three groups discussed "Parity, stigmatization and social participation" including one made up of individuals with mental disability (8 members), another with individuals with alcohol and drug problems (11 members), and a third of family members of individuals with mental disorders (7 members).

Theme A: Parity, stigmatization and societal participation

- In discussing attitudes and behaviours towards individuals with physical disorders, mental disorders and alcohol- and drug-related disorders, the participants considered that the latter two were more stigmatized than the first. Of the latter two, mental disorders are less stigmatized than alcohol- and drug-related disorders. Participants felt that the family is generally supportive towards subjects with mental and alcohol- and drug-related disorders, but with time attitudes change to neglect and even hate. Individuals with alcohol- or drug-related disorders are castigated by neighbours and workmates, with the result that they hide their problems. The marriage prospects of individuals with ADM disorders often suffer and their children and spouses are often stigmatized.

- Awareness of existing laws and social programmes was poor among participants in all the categories. Physically disabled persons and their family members were more aware than the mentally disabled and their family members. Awareness of tax relief and other financial benefits and knowledge of equal opportunities in employment were absent.

- Differences in attitude were considered to be dependent on the severity of the behaviour ral disturbances in the mental disorders category: the more severe these disturbances, the greater the stigmatization.

- The participants – including individuals with mental disorders and alcohol- and drug-related disability and their family members – felt that the laws were equal for both these groups and persons with physical disability, but that far more services were provided for the latter. Facilities such as soft loans and concessional tickets were available for the physically disabled.

Theme B: Current practices and needs

- Subjects with physical disability and family members of physically disabled persons had poor knowledge of the laws on disability. Even the latest act, enacted in 1996, had not been heard of by the majority of participants. Awareness of governmental programmes was also poor, though there was some knowledge of facilities provided such as concessional tickets, preferential housing allotments and telephone connections, and so forth. The availability of free appliances and treatment provided by the government was known, but only to a few. Professional care-givers were aware of these facilities. Most focus group members were not aware of the private and NGO-based programmes, though the health professionals knew of them.

- Health professionals knew the procedure to receive services. The cumbersome process and urban-rural inequality were often discouraging.

- The participants felt that free medical treatment, provision of aids and appliances, and other services should be made available by the government and that socioeconomic status and the severity of the disability should be the guiding principles for services.

- The view that the family should be the primary care provider for individuals was unanimous. The community and government should assist the family in carrying out its duties towards the disabled. The rapid change in community organization was, however, felt to hamper a clear definition of the community's role in taking care of disabled individuals.

- Lack of awareness of treatment facilities, lack of follow-up after treatment, and differential quality of treatment facilities were some of the gaps according to the participants.

- Changes mentioned as necessary for better management of individuals with disabilities were: improving facilities, including medical, rehabilitative and social facilities; changes in the physical environment to make it more disabled-friendly; making society more aware of the potential of disabled individuals; greater professional commitment; and introduction of educational, vocational and rehabilitation programmes.

Conclusion

Physical disorders have long been recognized as a leading cause of disability in India as elsewhere in the world, despite the general dearth of literature on the subject. However, there is now a growing awareness of mental disorders as a major reason for disability. The Global Burden of Disease study (Murray & Lopez 1997) estimated that depression was the fourth largest cause of disability-adjusted life years (DALYs) globally. The relationship between depression and disease burden has been emphasized in a global as well as Indian context in a recent editorial (Saxena & Dhawan 1999). Another study (Reinhard & Horwitz 1995) that assessed the family burden in 163 family members of 200 severely mentally ill subjects about to be discharged found high levels of both objective and subjective burden.

Other psychiatric disorders responsible for high disease burden are alcohol use, schizophrenia, bipolar affective disorders and obsessive compulsive disorder (Andrews, Sanderson & Beard 1998). The literature on disability and burden from India supports the literature available from elsewhere. One study from Chennai (formerly Madras) using the Schedule for the Assessment of Psychiatric Disability (SAPD) (Thara, Rajkumar & Valecha 1988) showed a relatively stable deficit in the 4th–6th year of illness, though there was much more disability in the acute stages (Thara & Raj Kumar 1993). The burden was markedly greater in family members who dealt with patients showing disruptive behaviour in this study.

Other studies from India have compared patients with schizophrenia and patients with mood (affective) disorders with regard to family burden, dysfunction and subjective well-being (Roychoudhari et al. 1995; Chakrabarti et al., 1995). These studies showed that the burden experienced is greater in family members of patients with schizophrenia. In a study on depression (Chadda 1995) no correlation was found between dysfunction and the social support patients received. The limited literature thus indicates greater disability and dysfunction in major psychiatric disorders, though definite conclusions cannot be drawn. Reliable estimates as to the overall extent of the problem of disabilities are not available. However, a report presented at a national seminar on rural rehabilitation at Nasrapur (Sethi 1980) put the figure for handicapped children at 3–9 million. Current estimates suggest that the prevalence of disability is 5% and the total affected population is approximately 50 million.

Another issue that has an important relationship to societal attitudes to disability is the legal situation in the country. In recognition of the growing global awareness, the Indian Parliament recently enacted the *Persons with Disabilities Act, 1996*, which shows the nation's concern to tackle issues related to disability. However, it appears that awareness of this progressive act is still limited.

The ICIDH-2 cross-cultural applicability research involved assessments using standard procedures and informants encompassing individuals with disability, family members of individuals with disability, health care providers, policy-makers, and others.

It appeared from the interviews and the centre description that, despite India's large population of individuals with disability, recognition of these individuals is rare and policies till recently included only those with physical disorders and mental retardation. It is only with the recent *Persons with Disabilities Act, 1996* that other disorders – particularly mental disorders – have been included. It is a progressive act, providing accommodations and opportunities far in excess of what were previously available. The implementation and awareness of the Act, however, are uniformly poor. A daily newspaper recently noted that the provisions of the Act are openly flouted in recruiting individuals for jobs in various governmental and nongovernmental agencies.

Each state is responsible for providing compensation and financial aid to people with disabilities. There is an elaborate system for measuring the physical disability for compensation. Various institutions, notably the Armed Forces, have clearly defined guidelines for compensation.

The results of the linguistic analysis showed certain difficulties in translation of the ICIDH-2 terms into Hindi, the national and local language, and these difficulties were noted in various points of the translations. However, most of the concepts in list A and list B could be easily transferred into Hindi. "Disability" was difficult to translate and "use of humour" when translated does not have the same wide implication as the original term.

Considerable overlap existed in the use of "impairment," "disability" and "participation." Disapproval ratings showed similar results in key informants interview when compared with All India ratings. There was a high degree of tolerance of disability in general, but disability related to mental disorders and alcohol and drug abuse is not well tolerated. Public reaction is strongest for facial disfigurement, use of drugs and use of alcohol, and least for intellectual slowness. There was a high degree of tolerance to behaviours exhibited by mentally ill, mentally subnormal and physically disabled people. It was felt that barriers to carrying out various activities would not generally be encountered.

The concept mapping exercise picked out certain items that were felt not to be culturally congruent, for example dating. Some were also felt to be inappropriate depending on age, gender or socio-economic status. The pile sorting exercise produced 13 distinct clusters.

The focus group discussions threw significant light on the perceptions of the various participants on parity, stigmatization, and societal participation and on current practices and needs. The group considered that there was discrimination, through perception differed across the categories of participants. In general, ADM disorders were more discriminated against than physical disorders. Similarly, facilities, including compensation, were better for the latter disorders. Disability related to drug use disorder was the most discriminated against, in all spheres of functioning. There was poor awareness of existing facilities, and when available they were not sufficiently utilized. Overall there seemed to be a growing awareness of issues related to disability.

Chapter 10
Japan

*M. Tazaki and Y. Nakane**

Highlights from the CAR study in Japan

- In Japan, attitudes towards the disabled have become more positive over the last few years.
- New plans for social welfare services and the structural reform of the social security system are now being implemented in an effort to adapt to an ageing society.
- Disabilities associated with physical, mental, and alcohol and drug disorders are still strongly discriminated against.
- There is a considerable felt need for improvement in the facilities, services and opportunities for the disabled.
- Participation of persons with disabilities in society needs to be promoted more vigorously.
- The model of disability in ICIDH-2 may need some culturally specific modification if it is to be acceptable to people with disabilities and the public in Japan.

Introduction

As a result of a rapid economic growth Japan has been the world's second largest market economy since 1993 (UNDP 1993). Concomitantly, the life expectancy of the Japanese people became the highest in the world for both sexes (males, 77.19 years; females, 83.82 years) in 1997 (Ministry of Health and Welfare 1997), probably because of the high standard of living and a

---
* Science University of Tokyo (Tazaki); Nagasaki University, School of Medicine (Nakane), Japan.

nationwide health care system. It is expected that the percentage of people over 65 years old in Japan will reach more than 25% of the population by the year 2000 (Ministry of Health and Welfare 1999). Consequently, the social security system has had to be reformed to integrate medical care with welfare. In addition to Japan's social welfare system, several targeted plans (the Gold Plan, the Angel Plan and the Plan for People With Disabilities) have been formulated and scheduled for adoption. The structural reform of the social security system of long-term care insurance will come into effect during the year 2000 (Ministry of Health and Welfare 1999).

Social welfare system

Japan's social welfare system consists of four major components: public assistance, social insurance, social welfare services, and public health maintenance. *Public assistance* is designed to assure a minimum level of security to those who are unable to earn a subsistence-level income. *Social insurance* consists of four main areas: health and medical insurance, public pensions, unemployment insurance, and workers' compensation. *Public health maintenance* includes public sanitation and the prevention and treatment of infectious diseases. There are three major types of *social welfare services:* services for the disabled, services for the aged, and services for children. Programmes for the disabled persons include pensions, institutional care, rehabilitation programme, special education, cash subsidies, medical counselling and home helper programme.

The Gold Plan was established in 1994 to promote health care and welfare for the elderly, including long-term care service. The Golden Plan will shortly replace this plan. The Angel Plan was established to promote support for child rearing and to enhance the total fertility rate which has fallen steadily in Japan for the past two decades. The Plan for People With Disabilities was established in 1995 with the aim of achieving rehabilitation and normalization (integration) in the community at all stages of life, for all forms of disability.

The CAR study was conducted while these reforms were being discussed and designed. Over the last few years, high unemployment due to economic recession has produced a fear of the future among many people in Japan. This has been accompanied by a change in both positive and negative attitudes towards the elderly and persons with disabilities. The results of the CAR study reflect the change in attitudes and the differences of opinion about disabilities found in Japan at this time.

Location of the study

The study was conducted mainly in Nagasaki and Tokyo, with the cooperation of health professionals and care-givers. Participating programme included the School of Medicine, Nagasaki University, and Tokyo Metropolitan Wakaba Welfare Centre for mental disability, Japan College of Welfare, St. Mariannan University, Tama Kyuryo Hospital, Teikyo University and Tokai University for physical disability, and the National Simousa Rehabilitation Centre, the Self-help Drug Rehabilitation Centre, Kanto-koshinetsu Regional National Narcotic Control Office and Fuchu Prison for alcohol and drug addiction.

The data were gathered from January to April in 1997 and recorded for analysis at the Science University of Tokyo. The results were then sent to Geneva to be analysed and compared with data from the rest of the participating centres.

Methods

The Japan site completed all basic components of the CAR study: the focus groups (the reports of focus groups were excluded here for reasons of space), linguistic analysis, key informant interviews followed by the self-administered questionnaire, and pile sorting and concept mapping.

Instruments

Linguistic analysis

The linguistic analysis followed the WHO translation guidelines and linguistic analysis protocol. The ICIDH-2 draft was translated into Japanese, any problems in translation being noted and attended to. Then the two lists of linguistic problem terms were translated from the original English into Japanese by a bilingual person. Two health professionals and two lay persons with minor disabilities were asked to identify any inadequately translated or unfamiliar words in the lists. Once the lists were deemed correct, back-translation was conducted by a different linguistic expert at Nagasaski University. The process was then repeated, since several terms from the original list were found to be inconsistent. After a couple of revisions, the translation of the materials was completed. This turned out to be a difficult task, because some of the technical terms – jargon – and some of the abstract words in the problem term lists were unfamiliar to both the translators and the persons with disabilities. A great deal of time was expended in revising concepts that did not seem to match exactly the terms or concepts that Japanese people would use in a given context.

Pile sorting and concept mapping

The pile sorting was conducted by writing a standardized set of 90 concepts and a brief definition on cards, and asking respondents to place them in piles of items that fitted together. The WHO pile sorting protocol was followed for data collection and recording. The 90 items for both the pile sorting and concept mapping were translated from English into Japanese using the WHO translation protocol. The concept mapping questionnaire (90 items plus definitions and 10 questions about each item) were administered to the recommended sample of respondents.

Key informant interview

The self-administered questionnaire for the key informant interviews was also first translated into Japanese by a professional translator. Terms and the wording of the questions were checked for comprehensibility, and back-translated in the same way as for the pile sorting and concept mapping.

Participants

Pile sorting and concept mapping

A total of 21 participants (13 males and 8 females) were selected to complete both exercises, pile sorting and concept mapping. The sample included 14 professionals and 7 patients; 4 professionals and 2 patients were drawn from alcohol and drug programmes; 2 professionals and 4 patients and care-givers from physical disability programmes; and 8 professionals and 1 patient from mental disability programmes. The mean age of the participants was 39.5 years old. Because of the length of the instruments, six participants were not able to complete the whole set of instruments, and these data were excluded.

Key informant interviews

A total of 18 participants (17 males and 1 female), consisting of 13 professionals and 5 care-givers and patients, were selected for the key informant exercise. The professionals included the best possible informants in Japan.

Out of 13 professionals, 3 were selected from the drug and alcohol field; 4 from the field of physical disability; and 6 from the field of mental disability. The mean age of the participants was 47 years. All the participants were recruited using targeted cultural expert sample selection procedures.

Procedures

All the interviews were conducted by the interviewers at the participants' workplace or home. No payment was given for participation in the study. There were four interviewers at the Tokyo site and two interviewers in Nagasaki. Prior to the interview, the purpose and procedure of the study were explained, and the participants were asked whether they agreed to participate in the study. Following the consent procedure, the interviewer completed the respondent face sheet. Patients were asked to sign a consent form for participation in the study.

The key informant interviews were tape-recorded and notes were taken by the interviewer. Following the interview, participants were asked to complete the self administered questionnaire. Some of them preferred to complete it later, by themselves, because of the length of the questionnaire; in such cases the interviewer gave them a pre-stamped envelope to send it by mail to the coordinator. Finally, they completed the rank-order task, using 16 cards pre-typed with the titles of disabilities.

For the pile sorting, after giving instructions and describing the instruments, the researcher placed the cards in front of the participants. The participants were then asked to place cards in piles as they wished. After the task was completed, the researcher asked the reason for each pile and its title. Once the pile sorting exercise was completed, a self-administered questionnaire was given to the participants, and all of them were asked to forward it to the coordinator by mail using a pre-stamped envelope.

Results

Linguistic analysis

The respondents completed the analysis of the 44 items included in list A. Generally speaking, most of the items were easily translated into Japanese and were both culturally and linguistically acceptable.

However, several words were found to present some type of problem of cross-cultural applicability. These are described below.

1. The concepts of impairment, disability, and handicap were not clearly distinguishable in Japanese, so only one word, *shogai*, was used to translate each of these three words. *Shogai* is an umbrella word that covers the concept of all three words.

2. Some of the concepts were difficult to translate because there is no equivalent term in Japanese, such as "executive functions." These concepts had to be explained.

3. The concepts that did not back-translate properly included "perception," "civic and community life," and "affect." These words are not found in Japanese and had to be explained.

Key informant interview and self-administered questionnaire

Qualitative analysis

The information in the key informant interviews revealed that a single word, *shogai*, was used to describe three concepts – impairment, disability, and handicap – in Japanese. The English differences are not captured by different words and have to be explained in some other way.

The interviews showed a difference in the ways that disabilities are treated in society. In all cases, it was true that physically disabled persons would have a hard time to find a job, or get married. In some cases people would feel sympathy for them. However, if the disabilities came from birth defects or were caused by a road accident, they were sometimes considered to come from family traits, as punishment for misbehaviour in a previous life as the consequence of the negative actions of family members, or from bad luck. In these cases, the disabilities were seen as punishment , not deserving sympathy. People with alcohol and drug problems, were considered to have problems because of their weak will power, and were felt not to deserve compensation, though they should be treated properly.

Quantitative analysis

Stigma rating. Eighteen health conditions were rated in terms of stigma. The three least stigmatizing conditions were being obese, being unable to read, and facial disfigurement. The three most stigmatizing were drug addiction, chronic mental retardation, and HIV-positivity as shown in Table 1.

Table 1. Social disapproval (stigma rating) ˙

Health condition	Mean	SD	Number of respondents
Obesity	2.06	1.06	16
Inability to read	3.75	2.29	16
Facial disfigurement	3.81	1.97	16
Cannot hold a job	3.88	1.31	16
Wheelchair-bound	4.31	2.52	16
Does not take care of own children	4.37	2.22	16
Borderline intelligence	4.40	2.35	16
Dirty and unkempt	4.56	2.22	16
Blind	4.88	2.60	16
Dementia	5.19	2.51	16
Leprosy	5.25	2.65	16
Homeless	5.81	2.71	16
Criminal record for burglary	5.94	2.93	16
Alcoholism	6.25	2.27	16
Depression	6.75	2.59	16
HIV-positive	6.87	2.75	16
Chronic mental disorder	7.13	2.20	16
Drug addiction	7.67	2.19	16

Public reaction ratings. Ten conditions were presented to the respondents. The three that elicited the least negative reactions in Japanese society were someone with a disfigured face, a woman in her eighth month of pregnancy, and someone who is blind. The three most negative reactions were directed at someone who is intellectually slow, someone with a chronic mental disorder who acts out, and someone who is visibly drunk.

In our society, public problems of drug addiction have not yet come significantly to the surface. The participants told us that they had never seen drug addicts on the street, so they could not evaluate the stigma of that condition. The three least stigmatized conditions were someone with a face disfigured by burns, a woman in her eight month of pregnancy, and someone who is blind (see Table 2).

Rank-order of disability. Of 17 disabling conditions, the three most disabling conditions were considered to be dementia, quadriplegia, and total blindness. The least three disabling conditions were: vitiligo on the face, infertility and mild mental retardation, as described in Table 3.

Activities. The average rating of the likelihood that "people would be surprised if the persons did this activity" across all 10 activities was calculated for each of the five health conditions. The order of the condition which elicited the least to the most surprise were a person in a wheelchair was a person

Table 2. Public Reaction % percentage of participants that rank the box

Condition	No issue/ no attention	Notice/ no issue	Uneasy	Uneasy/ avoid	Wrong/ say something	Wrong/ try to stop it
Someone with chronic mental disorder who acts out		6.3%	25.0%	56.3%	6.3%	6.3%
A woman in 8th month of pregnancy		93.8%	6.3%			
A person in a wheelchair		50.0%	43.8%	6.3%		
A person who is intellectually slow		7.7%	23.1%	46.2%	23.1%	
Someone who is dirty and unkempt	6.3%	31.3%	37.5%	25.0%		
Someone with a face disfigured by burns	18.8%	75.0%	6.3%			
An obese person	3.3%	31.3%	6.3%	37.5%	18.8%	
Someone who is visibly drunk		18.8%	31.3%	43.8%	6.3%	
Someone who is visibly under the influence of drugs						
Someone who is blind		12.5%	50.0%	37.5%		

Table 3. Ranking of disabilities

Health condition	Rank	Mean	SD	Number of respondents
Dementia	1	13.67	3.66	18
Quadriplegia	2	13.22	4.91	18
Total blindness	3	12.22	3.06	18
Paraplegia	4	11.72	2.30	18
Active psychosis	5	11.11	4.73	18
Total deafness	6	10.94	2.62	18
Major depression	7	9.78	4.33	18
Below-the-knee amputation	8	9.39	4.53	18
Drug dependence	9	9.19	3.94	18
Rheumatoid arthritis	10	8.33	4.34	18
Alcoholism	11	7.61	4.17	18
HIV-Positivity	12	6.89	5.32	18
Incontinence	13	6.44	3.54	18
Severe migraines	14	6.06	3.80	18
Mild mental retardation	15	5.94	3.04	18
Infertility	16	5.06	4.80	18
Vitiligo on face	17	3.11	3.12	18

with alcohol problems, a person who hears voices, a person born with low intelligence, and someone with a heroin problem.

The order from least to most impact among the health conditions by average rating of the likelihood that "people would place restrictions or barriers on the person" was a person in a wheelchair, someone with alcohol problems, a person born with low intelligence, a person who hears voices, and someone with a heroin problem.

Concept mapping data

Almost all the participants complained of the length of the questionnaire and its repetitious content.

The concept mapping responses indicated a significant number of cross-cultural applicability problems with the 90 concepts. In part, this may have been caused by the Japanese translation of the questionnaire. According to the response data from the questions on clarity of the words and concepts, the respondents indicated that all of the words had clarification problems. The Japanese translation of questions 1 and 2 asked if it would be better if they were further clarified, rather than focusing on problems in the clarification. It appears that there are significant differences in the ways that the respondents would place the terms in categories in comparison with their placement in ICIDH. In response to question 9, only nine words would have been placed in the same categories as they are in the draft ICIDH-2.

The items for which more than 25% of the participants reported problems are listed in Table 4.

Table 4. Problematic items for more than 25% of participants

Not useful for all age groups	Religious activity
	Work acquisition and retaining behaviours
	Performing consensual sexual acts
Not useful for all social economic groups	Using special means of communication
Not useful for ethnic/minority groups	Using special means of communication
	Using public transport
	Religious activity
Culturally sensitive	Activities related to fulfilling of financial obligations and services
	Cooking, baking, frying solid foods as part of cooking a meal
	Religious activity
	Sexual functions

Pile sorting

Based on a Johnson's hierarchical cluster analysis dendrogram using pile sorting data, 17 clusters were formed at the cut-off point of 0.3951. Each cluster and domain name is displayed in Table 5, in which items with an asterisk showed a strong central tendency to be associated with core items, and items with a minus sign were the least strongly associated with other items. The domain names use the titles of the central items. These are items that either were associated with multiple clusters during the pile sort process, or were sometimes seen as isolate or difficult to classify with the other items.

Table 5. Number of items included in each cluster

Cluster	Domain name	Cluster composition
1	Dating activities	77-, 71*, 83*
2	Sensory function	3-, 19, 25*, 26*
3	Perception and recognition	5-, 44, 4, 7, 13, 21*, 60*
4	Affect	29, 57
5	Learning activities	34-, 9*, 59*
6	Communication	18, 8, 61, 55, 20*, 64*, 69-
7	Emotional expression	54-, 68, 49*, 85*
8	Body-related behaviour	6-, 1, 45, 56*, 66*, 53, 75
9	Eating activity	63-, 30, 51, 67*, 70*
10	Self-care	36-, 28*, 32, 42, 24, 10, 78
11	Work and economic self-sufficiency	17, 82
12	Cultural activity	58-, 52*, 73*
13	Interpersonal skills	14-, 23, 31, 35, 12*, 37*, 47, 86
14	Following instructions	76-, 48*, 79*
15	Civic and community	2*, 22*, 39, 89-
16	Sustained interaction	62, 88
17	Managing threatening situations	33, 90

Each cluster and the relationships among the items which form the cluster are identified below:

Cluster 1: Dating activities (3 items)
  77   Sexual functions
  71*   Dating and forming a sexual relationship
  83*   Performing consensual sexual acts
Cluster 2: Sensory function (4 items)
  3   Seeing
  19   Visual sensory function

25* Hearing
26* Hearing functions

Cluster 3: Perception and recognition (7 items)
5   Attention
44   Consciousness
4   Memory
7   Thought, abstraction, judgement, and related executive functions
13   Recognizing directions in space and time
21* Perception
60* Recognizing

Cluster 4: Affect (2 items)
29   Temperament and personality
57   Affect

Cluster 5: Learning activities (3 items)
34   Citizenship responsibilities
9*   Acquiring and applying knowledge
59* Study behaviours

Cluster 6: Communication (7 items)
18   Non-verbal means of communication
8   Using special means of communication
61   Written communication
55   Communication activities
20* Use of communication life
64* Communication content
69   Abilities related to learning

Cluster 7: Emotional expression (4 items)
54   Use of humour
68   Conversation processes and structure
49* Expressing empathy
85* Responding to conversational cues

Cluster 8: Body-related behaviour (7 items)
6   Mobility
1   Transferring oneself
45   Moving around
56* Changing a body position
66* Maintaining a body position
53   Handling technical devices/aids for locomotion
75   Handling body-attached technical aids

Cluster 9: Eating activity (5 items)
63   Taking care of pets/domestic animals

30   Eating and drinking
51   Planning/organizing meals
67*   Cooking, baking, frying solid
70*   Taking care of meals

Cluster 10: Self-care (6 items)
36   Handling everyday physical environment
28*   Taking care of one's health
32   Maintaining physical environment
42   Self-care
24   Keeping oneself clean and appropriately groomed
10   Dressing
78   Washing oneself

Cluster 11: Work and economic self-sufficiency (2 items)
17   Economic self-sufficiency
82   Work acquisition and retention behaviour

Cluster 12: Cultural activity (3 items)
58   Following events that take place outside the direct environment
52*   Cultural activities
73*   Religious activities

Cluster 13: Interpersonal skills (8 items)
14   Keeping appropriate physical contact, and maintenance of social space
23   Showing tolerance in relationships
31   Interpersonal and social relationships
35   Managing close personal relationships
12*   Interacting with an equal/co-worker/peer
37*   Managing relationships with friends
47   People sharing living place
86   Taking care of household or family members

Cluster 14: Following instructions (3 items)
76   Keeping rules, abiding by decisions
48*   Following written instruction
79*   Following verbal instructions

Cluster 15: Civic and community (4 items)
2*   Community
22*   Civic and community life
39   Citizenship responsibilities
89   Using public transport

Cluster 16: Sustained interaction (2 items)
62   Managing general psychological demands

88   Managing personal behaviour

Cluster 17: Managing threatening situations (2 items)
33   Managing a dangerous environment
90   Responding to dangers

Some concepts could be classified within clusters, but showed only marginal association with the clusters. This indicates that the placement of these items in the ICIDH-2 classification was problematic.

50   Problem-solving
81   Language
38   Motor coordination
15   Leisure
16   Understanding specific signs
65   Activities related to fulfilling of financial obligations and services
87   Monitoring and evaluation of performance of activities/tasks

Within cluster 8: (Getting around), items 53 and 75 formed a marginal subgroup within the cluster. Similarly, within cluster 10, two independent subgroups could be distinguished. The first one consisted of items 28, 32 and 42; the second, items 24, 10 and 78.

The strongest cluster was Cluster 15 (Interpersonal skills), in which the level of association of all the concepts in the cluster was greater than 0.7309. The results of the clusters seem to fit well with the ICIDH-2 classification and in most cases match the placement of the items within the classification.

Conclusion

The CAR was successful in investigating and describing the current situation that people with disabilities face in Japanese society. The focus groups (not included here) provided an excellent introduction to the issues of discrimination and stigma faced by the persons with disabilities, and the challenges facing the health professionals and care-givers who assist them. The quantitative methods and the translation and linguistic analysis protocol revealed a number of discrepancies in concept, definitions, and phrasing of the draft ICIDH-2 which need to be corrected to make the classification cross-culturally applicable in Japanese society.

The linguistic analysis demonstrated that most of the words in lists A and B were transferable into Japanese. However, participants in the other exercises often asked for clarification of concepts and for a clear definition of the words used. Terms for a number of concepts could be found in Japanese, but their usage in the classification did not fit match the way they are used in daily life. Therefore, more clarification of the definition of uncommon words is recommended. The results also indicated that technical jargon should be excluded wherever possible.

In addition, the translation process identified some sentences that were unclear in the original English. This made translated sentences equally unclear. It is recommended that the sentences identified be rewritten in clear English, so that they can be correctly translated.

The key informant interviews revealed that social disapproval and public reaction are common for all kinds of disabilities. People with physical disabilities are not given much chance of employment or of getting marriage and having a family. Significant stigma is attached to all forms of disability. Thus it is a consistent finding that people would say something negative about a person appearing in public who is obese, or intellectually slow.

The concept mapping exercise identified several items which were problematic to use in our culture. In particular, items relating to religious and sexual activities caused serious reactions because of cultural taboos. The Japanese classification of the items into the levels of impairment, activity or participation was also found to differ greatly from the draft ICIDH-2. In part, this was felt to be the result of the lack of participation of people with disabilities in society, so that participation items were most often placed in the other two categories.

Conversely, the association of the items in the pile sort clusters was found to be similar to those in the draft ICIDH-2. However, the data still need an extended examination to identify the areas and rationale of both consensus and differences, in order to understand how the structure of the concepts in ICIDH-2 fit into our society.

In the Japanese welfare system, people with disabilities are provided with a variety of welfare services, which include pensions, cash subsidies, institutional care, special education and rehabilitation programme. They are assured a minimum level of subsistence, but stigma against them is still strong. Some families avoid receiving any benefits, because they are afraid of being publicly noticed as having a person with a disability in their home. They feel ashamed to have somebody disabled in the family. This feeling of shame appears to come from being identified as differing from the standard in the society – a common condition of "shame cultures," as Ruth Benedict (1934, 1977) pointed out some years ago. Historically, the Japanese have tended to lack public or institutional care for the elderly and the disabled because, as the weakest members of society, they were unable to be productive. Care was left to families to provide. However, as the society faces an ageing population, people have started to realize that the problems of the disabled will become their own problems in the near future when they themselves get older. Attitudes towards the disabled have changed positively to some extent over the last few years, and this is expected to lead to a society that provides more services for all, with or without any kind of disability, in the future.

Chapter 11
Luxembourg

C.B. Pull, A. Sztantics, J.M. Cloos, S. Muller, I. Heuertz, and M.C. Pull

Highlights from the CAR study in Luxembourg

- There remains a considerable need to improve and increase the services provided for all those who require them.
- Stigma continues to be more severe for mental disabilities than for physical disabilities.
- Families need relief from the pressures of dealing with the needs of persons with disabilities.

Introduction

Luxembourg is the smallest country in the European Community. Its standard of living is one of the highest, and unemployment rates are among the lowest (under 4%). The population of Luxembourg is about 410,000 (1995) with a density of 150 inhabitants/km²; almost 50% of the population live in rural areas. The largest urban centre is Luxembourg City, with some 100,000 inhabitants. The overwhelming proportion of people are white, Caucasian, and Roman Catholic. Only a small proportion of the people belong to other ethnic groups.

The health and social security systems of Luxembourg apply by and large to most of the population. The social security system is divided into a contribution level and a non-contribution level. The contribution level is directed to all workers who pay social security taxes. The non-contribution level is for people who have never reached the minimum salary established by law. The system provides coverage for all conditions, whether acute or chronic, physical or mental. For mental disorders, the social security system provides acute, long-term, and emergency treatment in psychiatric units. It provides rehabilitation and prevention programme for disabilities resulting from physical, mental,

---

* Centre Hospitalier de Luxembourg Service de Neuropsychiatrie, Luxembourg.

alcohol and drug disorders. "Disability tables" are used to define the degree of disability compensation for each type of disability. The extent of an injury determines the percentage disability for casualties, and those disabled after road or industrial accidents receive the most substantial economic support from the system. For mental disorders, compensation decisions are mainly based on the degree of handicap in social and professional function.

The presence and severity of disability are assessed primarily by physicians. A new law to provide additional assistance for disabled citizens (Assurance Dépendance) was introduced in 1998. The funds for this assistance are generated through a special tax which is paid by people in employment (1% of the monthly income). Family support is still very strong in Luxembourg society. A high proportion of persons with disabilities due to physical illnesses or mental disorders (e.g., persons with schizophrenia) are supported by their families, and many of them live with their close relatives.

Methods

Centre description

The CAR study relating to alcohol and drug use and mental (ADM) disorders was conducted as a joint project between the Luxembourg Centre de Recherche Public Santé (CRP-Santé), the World Health Organization, and the European Community (Biomed). The members of the research team in Luxembourg all belonged to the Psychiatric Department of the Centre Hospitalier de Luxembourg, a WHO Training and Reference Centre for the Mental Disorders Section of the Tenth Revision of the International Classification of Diseases (ICD-10), the Composite International Diagnostic Interview (CIDI), the Schedules for Clinical Assessment in Neuropsychiatry (SCAN), and the International Personality Disorders Examination (IPDE). The study was conducted in collaboration with the Centre Thérapeutique d'Useldange (Director P. Neuberg), the Centre Thérapeutique de Manternach (Director R. Pauly) and the Centre de Rééducation/Réadaptation Fonctionnelles de Hamm (Dr. G. Grenot). The data for the study were collected from February to May 1997, and the results were sent to Geneva to be analyzed and compared with those from the other participating countries.

Instruments and procedures

The Luxembourg site completed all the components of the CAR study.

Linguistic analysis

Two lists of terms related to disability – list A (44 items) and list B (67 items) – were translated into French, and then back-translated into English. The translation into French was done by bilingual experts in the field of disability, the back-translation by a French-English translator who was blind to the original English terms as well as to their translation into French.

Pile sorting

WHO proposed 90 items to be sorted into piles according to rules that were explained independently to each participant. The Luxembourg centre translated the terms, and printed each of them on individual cards. Each card included the name of an item and a brief definition. Each item was identified by a code number, printed on the back of the card.

Concept mapping

A hundred items, with their definitions, were translated into French. For each of these items, the participants were asked 10 questions concerning their acceptability in Luxembourg, their applicability according to sex, age and religion, and their relationship to the concepts of impairment, disability, and participation.

Key informant interviews

Key informant interviews consisted of three related exercises – an interview conducted by an interviewer, a self-administered questionnaire, and a ranking exercise – concerning a number of physical, mental, and alcohol- or drug-related disorders.

Focus groups

The Luxembourg centre conducted two focus groups, one with experts in the field of disability, the other with patients.

Sample

Participants were either professionals in the field of disability, or patients and care-givers. The linguistic analysis, pile sorting and concept mapping were done in two groups – a group of 15 professionals who were experts in the field of mental and physical health, and a group of 15 patients or care-givers of patients presenting with either a mental or a physical disorder. The key informant exercise was first completed with two groups, each of 15 par-ticipants, as described for the preceding tasks. In addition, the Luxembourg centre assembled a group of 80 mental health key informants, half of them professionals, the other half patients. Included in the patient group were 13 patients with a psychotic disorder, 15 with a recurrent mood disorder, 5 with an anxiety disorder, and 7 with alcohol or drug dependence. Included in the mental health professionals group were 10 medical professionals, 10 psy-chologists and psychiatric nurses 10, social workers and case-workers, and 10 policy-makers or opinion leaders. Participants in the "experts" focus groups included two medical doctors, two psychologists, two nurses, and two social workers. Participants in the "patients" group included two patients with a mental disorder, two with an alcohol disorder, two with a drug disorder, and two family members of patients with one of these disorders.

Results

Linguistic analysis

The majority of the items could be translated into French without any major difficulty. Items that raised problems are detailed in the following list:
1. Original English term: Disorder

    Translation into French: *Trouble*

    Back-translation into English: Trouble

The term *désordre* exists in French, meaning something that is not in order. The term is not generally used to designate an illness. In fact, how-ever, psychiatrists have begun to use the word *désordre* to refer to mental disorders, although it is not correct to use the French word in this context.
2. Original English term: Health condition

    Translation into French: *Etat de santé*

    Back-translation into English: State of health

There is no term in French to cover illnesses as well as conditions such pregnancy.
3. Original English term: Disablement

    Translation into French: *Handicap*

    Back-translation into English: Handicap

There is no umbrella term in French that covers "impairment," "disability," and "handicap."

4. Original English term: Well-being

   Translation into French: *Bien-être*

   Back-translation into English: Well-being

The French word does not convey the meaning of being in good health. It refers to feeling all right on a psychological level.

5. Original English term: Community

   Translation into French: *Communité*

   Back-translation into English: Community

The French word is not usually understood as referring to a close social environment. It pertains more to a broader concept, i.e., belonging to a certain social, ethnic or religious class.

Concept mapping

The concept mapping questionnaire revealed difficulties with the definitions provided for the following items: 4 (Memory); 6 (Mobility); 7 (Thought, abstraction, judgement); 8 (Special means of communication); 9 (Acquiring and applying knowledge); 12 (Interacting with an equal); 13 (Recognizing directions in space and time); 15 (Leisure); 30 (Eating and drinking); 39 (Citizenship responsibilities); 40 (Psychological endurance); 53 (Handling technical devices); 54 (Use of humour); 59 (Study behaviours); and 80 (Education). Another set of items were identified as not applying to all age groups: 17 (Self-sufficiency); 39 (Citizenship responsibilities); 42 (Self-care); 46 (Work); 51 Planning/organizing meals); 65 (Activities related to fulfilling financial obligations and services); 67 (Cooking, baking, frying solids); 76 (Keeping rules, abiding by decisions); 77 (Sexual function); 82 (Work acquisition); 83 (Performing consensual sexual acts); and 89 (Using public transport).

The following four items were identified as culturally sensitive: 14 (Keeping appropriate physical contact and maintenance of social space); 75 (Handling body-attached technical aids); 77 (Sexual functions); and 83 (Performing consensual sexual acts). Finally, there was considerable variation among participants as to the attribution of items to the three groups – impairments, disabilities or handicaps.

Pile sorting

One of the participants declined to do this exercise. The remaining 30 participants put the 90 items into 334 piles, ranging from as few as 3 piles to as many as 22, with a mean of 11 piles per participant. The results were included in the overall analyses carried out by WHO; no individual analyses on the Luxembourg data were done by the centre. However, the overall classification constructed from these data closely matches the ICIDH-2 classification, with the exception of the problematic items described above.

Key informant interviews and self-administered questionnaire

Analysis of the qualitative data in section A of the key informant questionnaire indicates that there is considerable overlap between different French words related to the concepts of disability and handicap. Key informants were not optimistic about the chances of persons with either a physical or a mental disorder getting a job, and even less so for persons with alcohol- or drug-related disorders. The general opinion in both focus groups was that patients with any of the disorders would encounter difficulties in getting married and having a family.

There was general agreement that patients with a physical disorder should be provided with social assistance as soon as possible. There was considerably less agreement concerning the type of social assistance from the government that should be provided to patients with a mental disorder or with disorders related to alcohol or drugs. The results obtained from the qualitative data in the group of patients with a psychotic disorder will be presented in more detail.

The answers from the open-ended questions were grouped, and the frequency of answers provided by professionals and patients is summarized in Table 1.

Table 1. Answers to open-ended questions on persons with a psychotic disorder (% of respondents)

Answers	Professionals (*n*=40)	Patients (*n*=40)	All (*n*=80)
First attracts attention by			
Psychomotor behaviour	55	31	44
Speech/communication	50	31	41
Appearance	10	5	8
None	13	23	18
Other	5	18	11

Some sign will attract attention			
If problem quite mild	87	77	82
If problem fairly serious	100	88	96
Signs that person needs help			
Psychomotor behaviour	65	55	60
Physical appearance	43	15	29
Speech/communication	10	5	8
Other	13	30	21
Affects work			
Very much	75	60	67
Somewhat	25	40	33
Affects marriage			
Very much	47	46	47
Somewhat	53	54	53
Should get social assistance			
Yes	58	55	56
No	8	20	14
Depends	33	20	27
Should get social assistance			
Immediately	25	23	24
After less than one month	5	0	3
After one month to one year	15	18	16
After more than one year	25	10	18
Other	30	49	39
Problems in daily activities			
Interpersonal relations	55	30	43
Occupational problems	28	25	26
Basic activities	28	25	26
Social isolation	43	35	39
If problem from birth			
More accepted	43	50	46
Less accepted	8	15	11
No effect	43	18	30
Other	6	17	13
If problem from accident			
More accepted	38	43	40
Less accepted	0	5	3
No effect	20	18	19
Depends on personal responsibility	25	25	25
Other	17	9	13

The first open-ended question was about aspects of the person's behaviour that might attract the attention or notice of others. With the exception of two patients, key informants agreed that a person presenting with psychotic symptoms would attract the attention of others, as soon as the problem was fairly serious. In addition, 87% of the professionals and 77% of the patients mentioned that persons with these types of symptoms would attract the attention of others even if their problem was only mild.

Abnormalities in behaviour, physical appearance and speech or communication were listed most frequently as the signs people would notice that a person with a psychotic disorder needed help from someone else to perform activities of everyday life. Abnormalities in psychomotor behaviour and in speech or communication were listed by 65% and 10% of the professionals and 55% and 5% of the patients. Abnormalities in physical appearance were listed significantly more often by professionals (43%) than by patients (15%).

In the opinion of 75% of the professionals and 60% of the patients, the problem would have a major impact on the person's ability to get work. 47% of the professionals and 46% of the patients said that the problem would greatly affect the person's ability to get married and have a family. According to the remaining key informants, a fairly serious problem of this sort would have at least some negative effect on the person's ability to get a job or do productive work, as well as to get married and have a family. Both professionals and patients listed difficulties in interpersonal relationships (55% vs 30%), social isolation (43% vs 35%), occupational problems (28% vs 25%), and problems in basic daily activities (28% vs 25%) as critical factors that would have an impact on everyday life.

About half of the participants (45% of the professionals and 41% of the patients) declared that people in their culture would propose that assistance from the Government should be granted within a year. An additional 25% of the professionals and 10% of the patients thought that people in their society would favour social assistance in such cases if the problem lasted more than one year. According to the answers of the remaining key informants (30% of the professionals and 49% of the patients), subsumed under "other," people in their society would favour assistance under certain conditions, e.g., if the problem was chronic or recurrent or if rehabilitation had been tried without success.

Most key informants (43% of the professionals and 50% of the patients) thought that people in their society would more easily accept a disability problem if it could be linked to a cause that had been present from birth. 38% of the professionals and 43% of the patients thought that people in their society would more easily accept a problem of this kind if it could be linked to a road accident. An additional 25% of the key informants said that the problem might be more easily accepted if the person had had no personal responsibility in the accident. According to 58% and 55% of the professionals and patients, people in their society would think that a person with this kind of problem should get social assistance from the government if the problem was serious. According to a further 33% and 20% of professionals and patients, entitlement to social assistance would depend on various factors, such as severity of symptoms or disability. Three professionals (8%) and 8 patients (20%) considered that people in their society would not favour any kind of assistance in such cases.

Table 2 presents the percentages of key informants indicating that people would be surprised (or very surprised) if a person hearing voices performed various activities, and that it would be likely (or very likely) that they would face barriers or restrictions in attempting to perform such activities.

Table 2. Likelihood that those in their culture would be surprised or very surprised if a person hearing voices performed the activity, and that barriers/restrictions would be placed on such a person (% of respondents)

Activity		Professionals ($n=40$)	Patients ($n=40$)	Total ($n=80$)
Keeping things tidy	Surprised	30	25	28
	Barriers/restrictions	28	28	28
Using public transportation	Surprised	18	18	18
	Barriers/restrictions	43	38	40
Being in love	Surprised	40	25	33
	Barriers/restrictions	58	55	56
Having sex (as part of a relationship with someone)	Surprised	38	23	30
	Barriers/restrictions	63	55	59
Actively taking on parenting roles	Surprised	80	65	73
	Barriers/restrictions	93	90	92
Actively taking part in community fairs and festivals	Surprised	33	40	36
	Barriers/restrictions	70	58	64
Managing own money	Surprised	38	40	39
	Barriers/restrictions	65	73	69
Getting an apartment or somewhere to live	Surprised	38	25	31
	Barriers/restrictions	65	60	63
Keeping a full-time job appointed	Surprised	60	55	58
	Barriers/restrictions	68	73	70
Being elected to a position in local government	Surprised	98	85	92
	Barriers/restrictions	100	90	95

A majority of both patients and professionals responded that people in their culture would be surprised or very surprised if such a person was appointed or elected to a position in local government, kept a full-time job, or took on parenting roles. In both groups, a minority of participants expressed surprise that such people might use public transportation, keep things tidy, be in love, have sex, can take active part in community fairs, manage their own money, or get an apartment. More professionals than patients volunteered that people in their culture would be surprised if such a person was in love, had a sexual relationship with someone, actively took on parenting roles, or got an apartment or somewhere to live, but none of these differences was statistically significant. With the exception of keeping things tidy and using public transportation, a majority of both professionals and patients considered that it was likely or very likely that people would place restrictions or barriers on the person if he or she wanted to perform any of the other activities. In particular, almost all the participants in both groups mentioned that it was likely or very likely that there would be such restrictions or barriers to being elected to a position in local government, actively taking on parenting roles, managing one's own money, keeping a full-time job, getting an apartment to live or somewhere to live, even taking part in community fairs. There were no statistically significant differences between the two groups of key informants for any of the items under investigation.

Rank order of 17 conditions

Respondents determined the relative rank order of 17 health conditions, ranked from most disabling to least disabling. There were no significant differences between the rankings by professionals and patients. Overall, active psychosis was considered the third most disabling condition, preceded only by quadriplegia and dementia. Both professionals and patients considered active psychosis more disabling than any physical disorder in the list, including blindness, paraplegia, deafness and HIV infection, as well as any other ADM disorder such as depression, drug addiction, alcoholism, and mental retardation. This is represented in Figure 1.

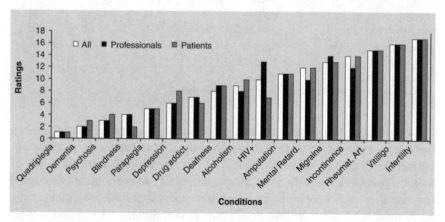

Figure 1. Disability rank-ordering from most disabling (lowest rank) to less disabling rank)

Ratings on social disapproval

The mean ratings of social disapproval are presented in Table 3, for the total sample and separately for the two groups of key informants. Mean ratings for social disapproval show that people who are blind, those in wheelchairs, and those with borderline intelligence meet with the least amount of social disapproval, while those with an alcohol problem, a criminal record for burglary, those who do not take care of their children and those with a drug problem receive the highest level of disapproval. The ratings on social disapproval place a person with chronic psychotic disorder on generally the same level as people who cannot hold down a job and those who suffer from leprosy or dementia.

Table 3. Ranking of degree of social disapproval/stigma by health condition

Health condition	All (n=80)			Professionals (n=40)			Patients (n=40)		
	Rank	Mean	SD	Rank	Mean	SD	Rank	Mean	SD
Blind	1	1.23	1.68	1	1.03	1.21	2	1.42	2.04
Wheelchair-bound	2	1.38	1.84	2	1.47	1.83	1	1.29	1.87
Borderline intelligence	3	3.12	2.28	3	3.03	2.34	3	3.21	2.24
Obese	4	3.16	2.24	4	3.00	1.71	4	3.32	2.66
Depression	5	3.61	2.22	6	3.56	1.98	5	3.66	2.45
Inability to read	6	3.89	2.68	5	3.64	2.59	7	4.13	2.78
Facial disfigurement	7	4.09	2.89	7	4.53	2.91	6	3.68	2.84
Cannot hold down a job	8	5.50	2.11	8	5.61	1.90	10	5.39	2.32
Chronic mental disorder	9	5.62	2.70	10	6.02	2.81	9	5.24	2.56
Leprosy	10	5.76	3.42	9	6.00	3.61	11	5.53	3.25
Dementia	11	5.91	2.98	11	6.14	3.04	8	5.68	2.95
Dirty and unkempt	12	6.69	2.52	12	6.64	2.37	14	6.74	2.69
Homeless	14	6.78	2.81	15	6.92	2.93	13	6.66	2.72
HIV-positive	13	6.97	2.59	13	6.64	3.05	12	7.29	2.05
Alcoholism	15	7.70	2.21	14	7.58	2.13	16	7.82	2.30
Criminal record for burglary	16	7.78	2.07	16	8.00	1.93	15	7.58	2.20
Does not take care of own children	17	8.01	2.10	17	8.03	2.08	17	8.00	2.16
Drug addiction	18	8.93	1.66	18	9.22	1.49	18	8.66	1.77

Ratings on public reaction

Table 4 presents the rank order of mean ratings of public reaction to persons with various health conditions appearing in public. Patients as well as professionals stated that people would pay attention when a person with a chronic mental disorder appeared in public. The majority of the participants (73%, comprising 80% of the professionals and 67% of the patients) indicated that people would feel uneasy when such a person appeared in public, e.g., on a bus or in a store or market. A proportion (15%) of the professionals as well as of the patients judged that people in their society would consider the presence of such patients in public places to be "wrong."

Table 4. Rating of public reaction to persons with 10 health conditions appearing in public (% of respondents).

Health Condition	All n=80			Professional n=40			Patients n=40		
	No issue	Un-easy	Wrong	No issue	Un-easy	Wrong	No issue	Un-easy	Wrong
1. A person in a wheelchair	59	41	0	65	35	0	52	48	0
2. Woman eight months pregnant	99	0	1	100	0	0	98	0	2
3. Someone who is blind	68	31	1	63	35	2	73	27	0
4. A person who is intellectually "slow"	46	53	1	43	57	0	50	48	2
5. Someone with a face disfigured from burns	35	59	6	30	63	7	40	55	5
6. An obese person	76	10	14	78	5	17	75	15	10
7. Someone with a chronic mental disorder	11	73	15	5	80	15	18	67	15
8. Someone who is dirty and unkempt	10	51	39	12	48	40	8	55	37
9. Someone who is visibly drunk	4	40	56	0	30	70	8	50	42
10. Someone who is visibly under the influence of drugs	3	41	56	0	40	60	5	42	53

Focus groups

The Luxembourg centre conducted two focus groups on current practices and needs in the field of disability. The first focus group was composed of professionals, the second of patients and care-givers. In both groups, participants were asked to answer and discuss the following items:

1. Description of programme available to persons with physical, mental health, and alcohol-and drug-related disabilities.

The two groups had difficulties with the term "programme," which is not generally used in this context. In Luxembourg more commonly used term is "services." Existing services for patients with ADM disorders include both inpatient and outpatient facilities, and rehabilitation services. Programme that offer help in the social reintegration of patients include services for both the physically and the mentally disabilities.

2. The process that someone must go through to become eligible to receive services and the responsibility of the government to provide assistance to persons with disabilities.

Opinions differed among participants as to whether this process should follow very stringent rules and procedures or whether it should be flexible, depending on each individual case. Participants agreed that the process depends on the patients' condition, but that it should not be rooted in too many rules. Rules that seemed acceptable to all participants included an initial check-up by a medical doctor, and detoxification in patients with alcohol or drug dependence syndrome. The participants emphasized the need for close collaboration between different services. Major problem areas include the lack of emergency services for patients with acute ADM disorders, the paucity of day-care centres for patients with Alzheimer's disease, and the paucity of day-care centres for patients with chronic psychotic disorders.

3. Responsibility of the family and community in providing services for persons with disabilities.

A majority of the participants agreed that substantial responsibility lies with the families of those who have a disability. In the groups' opinion, families should receive more help in providing services. Help from the government should be financial as well as psychological. Information about the services available should be more easily obtainable.

4. The gaps between services provided and services needed.

In both groups participants agreed that there is an urgent need for the creation or development of the following services; inpatient facilities for adolescents and elderly patients; inpatient treatment facilities for patients with eating disorders; outpatient facilities for patients with anxiety disorders and patients with psychosomatic disorders; and long-term facilities for patients with severe chronic psychotic disorders.

5. Changes needed to improve the conditions experienced by persons with mental and physical disabilities.

There was general agreement on the necessity to fight stigmatization of patients with any type of disability. In particular, participants favoured the adoption of programme to fight the stigma associated with schizophrenia and other mental disorders. In the participants' view, the single major change to be wished for in Luxembourg is a change in people's mind concerning patients with a handicap related to a physical or mental disorder.

Conclusion

Although a considerable number of facilities are at present available for patients presenting with a disability due to a physical, an alcohol- or drug-related, or a mental disorder, there is still a substantial need to improve and increase the services that should be provided for all those who require them.

Chapter 12
The Netherlands

*D. Van Hoeken, Y.F. Heerkens, M.W. De Kleijn-De Vrankrijker, and H.W. Hoek**

Highlights from CAR study in the Netherlands

- The Dutch have tolerance for people with various health conditions who appear in public, except in cases of "disturbing" behaviour, such as "acting out."

- People in The Netherlands tend to see health conditions of a permanent, incurable nature as very disabling. On the other hand, treatable health conditions and health conditions that can be concealed are considered less disabling.

- The high standard of state-provided facilities in The Netherlands means that there are few "objective" barriers to prevent people with a health condition from carrying out activities. However, particularly for people with low intelligence, social acceptability and likelihood of facing barriers are rated relatively less favourably.

- Even highly educated people working at policy making level have trouble in formulating the view of society on functioning and disability.

* Psychiatric Institute "Parnassia", WHO Collaborating Centre for the WHO/NIH Joint Project in The Netherlands (Van Hoeken; Hoek); Dutch National Institute of Allied Health Professions (Heerkens); WHO Collaborating Centre for the ICIDH in The Netherlands (Heerkens, De Kleijn-De Vrankrijker); TNO Prevention and Health (De Kleijn-De Vrankrijker); University of Leiden (Hoek), The Netherlands.

Introduction

The Dutch centre

The Dutch WHO Collaborating Centre for the WHO/NIH Joint Project on the Assessment and Classification of Disablements related to Alcohol and Drug Use and Mental (ADM) Disorders is based at the Parnassia Psychiatric Institute, The Hague, The Netherlands. It has a staff of nearly 3000, a capacity of over 1300 inpatient beds, and large day-care and outpatient facilities. The care is organized in six divisions: two adult psychiatry divisions, one of which is for chronic patients, two elderly (age 65 years and over) psychiatry divisions, one of which is for nursing care; an alcohol and drug division; and a youth (age below 18 years) psychiatry division. Parnassia serves an urbanized region of 500,000 inhabitants, including a growing number of legal and illegal immigrants. The largest groups of non-native inhabitants in the region are of Moroccan, Suriname, Turkish and Netherlands Antilles origin, but the current influx of refugees is coming mainly from Eastern European, Asian and African countries.

Dutch population data

The Netherlands is a small Western European country with a high population density (419 people per km²), yearly population growth of approximately 0.5%, and an increasing percentage of elderly people. By 1 January 1998 it had a population of 15,654,200 (7,740,100 men and 7,914,100 women). The age distribution was: 0–19 years, 24%; 20–39 years, 31%; 40–64 years, 31%; 65–79 years, 10%; and 80 years and over 3%. The mean age was 40 years. It is estimated that in the year 2010 11% of the population will be aged 65–79 and nearly 4% will be aged 80 and over (Central Bureau of Statistics, 1999).

The Netherlands is the eleventh wealthiest country in the Western world. The unemployment level is low, and both wages and the cost of daily living are high. Health facilities are well developed. There are about 775 centres for inpatient treatment, of which 80 are psychiatric institutes, and an average of 1.8 beds for psychiatry per 1000 inhabitants, including beds in psychiatric wards in general hospitals. There are extensive social support and educational systems. Education is obligatory and free of charge up to the age of 16.

Disability in The Netherlands

Compared to most other Western countries, the Dutch disability support system provides more income compensation and facilities for disabled people, through such means as the Disability Benefits Act (WAO), the Pension Fund for Civil Servants (ABP), and the General Disablement Pensions Act (AAW). Various other acts make special provision for the disabled, including the elderly. Vocational rehabilitation programmes, sheltered workplaces and special schools that include vocational training are also available for people with disabilities.

On the basis of a nationwide survey carried out in 1986–1988 it was estimated that in 1996 a total of 35% of the independently living persons aged 5 and over would have one or more physical disabilities. These ranged from minor to very severe, including 11.5% suffering from severe to very severe physical disabilities (Klerk & Timmermans 1998; Central Bureau of Statistics/Netherlands Institute for Research on Social Welfare 1990). It has been estimated that in 1995, 101,800 people in The Netherlands suffered from mental disabilities (Klerk & Timmermans 1998).

Methods

The Dutch site completed all the basic components of the CAR study: linguistic analysis, key informant interviews, followed by the self-administered questionnaire; pile sorting; and concept mapping. In addition, one focus group consisting mainly of mental health professionals was conducted. Five additional concepts were included in the concept mapping: dressing appropriately, incontinence, handling one's own social position/social responsibilities, low vision/binocular vision; and recognizing visual input.

Sample and procedures

Linguistic analysis

The translation from English into Dutch was done in two stages: after the initial translation by three experts, two other experts commented on the initial translation. The annotations and the questions for each item were also translated. For the translation back into English a list of 60 Dutch terms was compiled. The terms were arranged in alphabetical order.

Key informant interviews and self-administered questionnaire

Thirteen subjects were recruited using convenience sampling procedures. The respondents included health professionals and policy-makers, ADM health consumers and ADM care givers. The mean age of the key informants was 45 years. Six (46%) subjects were female. All professionals and policy-makers and opinion leaders had previously worked in the areas of physical disabilities and mental health, and most had also worked in the alcohol and drug field. The health consumers were selected for having long-standing impairments leading to considerable disability. The care-givers were selected for having long-term experience of caring for severely disabled people.

Prior to the interview, subjects were required to sign a consent form and complete a sheet of demographic questions. The interviews and questionnaires were conducted in Dutch.

Pile sorting

For the pile sort exercise 35 people were recruited: five psychiatric patients and 30 professionals with a vast range of experience in the field of psychiatry. The mean age was 35 years. Twenty-one subjects (60%) were male. The pile sorting was done in groups of 3–5 people. For each participant a set of cards was placed on a table as requested in the protocol. The text on the cards was in Dutch. Blank cards were available to write down the name of each pile and the reason for making the pile. The time available to perform the exercise was limited to 75 minutes.

Concept mapping

At the end of the pile sorting sessions the participants were asked to take part in the concept mapping as well. Of the 35 participants in the pile sort, 23 also participated in the concept mapping, of whom two were psychiatric patients. Twelve subjects were male (52%), one person did not note his or her gender. The mean age for the concept mapping was 37.

Each person received written instructions, the concept mapping questionnaire itself and an envelope in which to return the questionnaire. The written instructions and the concept-mapping questionnaire were both in Dutch.

Focus groups

The one focus group at the Dutch site was conducted with nine physicians. Although not all participants were familiar with the ICIDH model, all were familiar with the disability programme and beliefs about disabilities in the Dutch culture. The session was moderated by a discussant. After a short introduction, the views of the medical professionals on life domains important for people with a health condition were explored. A discussion was then held on the relevance and importance of the six life domains listed by WHO, and these six domains were evaluated relative to the domains proposed by the group. The focus group was held in Dutch.

Results

Linguistic analysis

At least five types of problems arose with the translation of English terms into Dutch and the back-translation of Dutch terms into English.

For a start, a one-to-one back-translation was difficult, as there are many Dutch terms that have a different meaning depending on the context. An example is the English term "community" which is normally translated by the Dutch term "*gemeenschap*." Back-translation into English out of context resulted in two different terms: "community" and "sexual intercourse."

Second, for some English terms there is only a more general term in Dutch. For instance, "disease" translates into Dutch as "*ziekte*." However, when translated back into English, "*ziekte*" becomes "illness" or "sickness." In a medical setting, illness indicates a specific, classifiable ailment. Sickness would indicate the actual state of being sick.

Third, for some English terms there are two or more specific Dutch terms. For instance, the English term "family" can be translated into the Dutch term "*familie*" and "*gezin*." The Dutch term "*familie*" indicates all relatives of a person, including grandparents, aunts, uncles, nieces, nephews, and so forth. The Dutch term "*gezin*" indicates a unit of people living together, most often father, mother and their (adopted) children. The English term "family" covers both "*familie*" and "*gezin*."

Fourth, for some English terms there is no Dutch equivalent term available. An example is the English term "disablement."

Finally, for some of the English terms it is better to choose a Dutch term with the same content than to use the official translation. For instance the Dutch term "*stoornis*" is a more neutral translation of the English term "impairment" than the official translation "*beschadiging*" or "*gebrek*," which is closer to the English term "disturbance." The Dutch term "*stoornis*" was therefore chosen as the most neutral general translation for the English term "impairment" in the translation of the 1980 version of ICIDH.

Key informant interviews and self-administered questionnaire

Almost all the respondents had difficulty in providing general terms for health conditions in section A of the interview. In section B of the interview, a need was felt for anchoring both the degree of severity of the health condition and the degree of reduction in functioning. A solution might be to provide a scale for both. For both substance use problems the question on problems related to death of a relative was considered irrelevant. In general, the respondents were more positive about the self-administered questionnaire than about the interview, finding it interesting and challenging their way of thinking about the consequences of having a health condition.

Qualitative analysis

Qualitative analysis of the interviews revealed that the Dutch term "*handicap*" could refer simultaneously to impairment, activity limitation, and lack of participation; but most specifically to impairment. In Dutch society, no agreement has been reached on general terms for lack of activity or of participation due to a health problem. Employment opportunities for people with physical or mental problems are much reduced. People of low intelligence are seen as able to perform simple, adapted work, but there is a shortage of such jobs. Job opportunities for people with low intelligence were believed to depend on the person's capacity for independent functioning.

Opportunities for getting married and having a family were not a general problem for people with alcohol problems, because the majority of this group is above the marrying/childbearing age. The respondents did not agree with each other whether people with a physical problem were stigmatized. For people with a mental or drug problem, societal stigma and isolation are greater and opportunities for employment are reduced.

There are no legal barriers to social or financial assistance once it has been established that there is a physical or mental inability to earn one's living. However, bureaucratic barriers make it difficult for those with mental problems or low intelligence to find employment, and social barriers operate for those with substance use problems. Some respondents indicated that detoxification is a prerequisite for social assistance.

Disabilities from birth or resulting from a road accident were generally regarded as deserving sympathy. However, sympathy was time-limited in the case of alcohol-related problems, and drug abuse was not tolerated.

Quantitative analysis

Stigma ratings
Table 1 sets out the Dutch means of social disapproval for the 18 health conditions.

The mean scores are on a scale from 0 to 10, with 0 representing no social disapproval and 10 representing extreme social disapproval.

Table 1. Rank order of Dutch ratings of degree of social disapproval

Health condition	Mean	SD
Blind	1.1	1.8
Wheelchair-bound	1.9	2.0
Inability to read	2.5	1.5
Borderline intelligence	2.6	2.5
Dementia	3.6	2.6
Depression	3.7	1.5
Obese	4.1	2.4
Chronic mental disorder	4.9	2.4
Cannot hold down a job	5.1	1.9
Facial disfigurement	5.2	2.4
Leprosy	5.6	3.3
Dirty and unkempt	6.3	2.8
Known to be HIV-positive	7.2	1.6
Cannot take care of own children	7.2	1.2
Homeless	7.5	1.7
Alcoholism	7.9	1.4
Criminal record for burglary	8.4	2.4
Drug addiction	9.3	0.9

Public reaction ratings
Of the 10 conditions presented, the three considered to elicit the most negative reactions in Dutch society were: visibly under the influence of drugs, having a chronic mental disorder with acting out, and visibly drunk. The least negative reactions were reserved for a woman in her eight month of pregnancy, a person in a wheelchair, and someone who is blind.

Rank-order of disability
The three conditions perceived as most disabling were: active psychosis, dementia and quadriplegia. Least disabling were: vitiligo on the face, infertility, and incontinence.

Activities

The order of conditions from least likely to most likely to elicit surprise by doing activities was: alcohol problems, heroin problem, in a wheelchair, hearing voices, and born with low intelligence. Drug addiction rated highest on the stigma ratings. On this point the Dutch apparently make a difference between the more objective observation of what people with certain conditions are able to do and the more subjective valuation of the condition.

The order from least to most likely to face barriers was: in a wheelchair, alcohol problems, hearing voices, a heroin problem and born with low intelligence. The level of education in The Netherlands is high, and great emphasis is placed on it. This negatively affects the opportunities for people who cannot meet these high educational standards.

Pile sorting

The mean number of piles was 11, with a range of 4–29. Visual inspection of the icicle plots in Johnson's hierarchical cluster analysis revealed 11 clusters in the Dutch data (see Table 2).

Table 2. Grouping of items in Dutch and overall study data based on Johnson's hierarchical cluster analysis

	Item	Item name	Clusters from Dutch data										
Clusters from overall study data	No.		A	B	C	D	E	F	G	H	I	J	K
1	2	Community											
	15	Leisure											
	22	Civic and community life											
	39	Citizenship responsibilities											
	52	Cultural activities											
	58	Following (showing interest in) events that take place outside the direct environment											
	73	Religious activities											
2	12	Interacting with an equal/co-worker/peer											
	14	Keeping appropriate physical contact, and maintenance of social space											
	23	Showing tolerance in relationships											

Clusters from overall study data	Item No.	Item name	Clusters from Dutch data										
			A	B	C	D	E	F	G	H	I	J	K
	31	Interpersonal and social relationships		■									
	35	Managing close personal relationships		■									
	37	Managing relationships with friends		■									
	47	People sharing living space		■									
	71	Dating and forming relationships		■									
	76	Keeping rules, abiding by decisions		■									
	77	Sexual functions		■									
	83	Performing consensual sexual acts		■									
3	17	Economic self-sufficiency			■								
	46	Work			■								
	65	Activities related to fulfilling of financial obligations and services			■								
	82	Work acquisition and retention behaviours			■								
4	10	Dressing				■							
	24	Keeping self clean and appropriately groomed				■							
	27	Organizing daily routine				■					■		
	28	Taking care of one's health				■							
	30	Eating and drinking				■							
	32	Maintaining physical environment				■							
	36	Handling everyday physical environment				■	■						
	42	Self-care				■							
	51	Planning/organizing meals				■							
	63	Taking care of pets/domestic animals				■							
	67	Cooking, baking, frying solids				■							
	70	Taking care of meals				■							
	78	Washing oneself				■							
	84	Procurement and care of necessities				■							

Clusters from overall study data	Item No.	Item name	Clusters from Dutch data										
			A	B	C	D	E	F	G	H	I	J	K
	86	Taking care of household or family members					■						
	87	Monitoring and evaluation of performance of activities, tasks					■				■		
5	1	Transferring oneself						■					
	6	Mobility						■					
	38	Motor coordination						■					
	45	Moving around						■					
	53	Handling technical devices/aids to locomotion						■					
	56	Changing a body position						■					
	66	Maintaining a body position						■					
	75	Handling body-attached technical aids						■					
	89	Using public transport						■					
6	8	Using special means of communication							■				
	16	Understanding specific signs							■				
	18	Non-verbal means of communication							■				
	20	Use of communication devices							■				
	48	Following written instructions							■				
	54	Use of humour		■					■				
	55	Communication activities involving at least two active participants							■				
	61	Written communication							■				
	64	Communication content							■				
	68	Conversation processes and structure		■					■				
	79	Following verbal instructions							■				
	81	Language							■				
	85	Responding to conversational clues						■					
7	9	Acquiring and applying knowledge								■			
	34	Arithmetic activities								■			
	50	Problem-solving								■			
	59	Study behaviours								■			
	69	Abilities relating to learning and communication								■			

Clusters from overall study data	Item No.	Item name	Clusters from Dutch data										
			A	B	C	D	E	F	G	H	I	J	K
	80	Education						■					
8	3	Seeing							■				
	11	Experience of pain							■				
	19	Visual sensory functions							■				
	25	Hearing							■				
	26	Hearing functions							■				
9	4	Memory							■				
	5	Attention							■				
	7	Thought, abstraction, judgement, and related executive functions							■				
	13	Recognizing directions in space and time							■				
	21	Perception							■				
	41	Orientation							■				
	43	Intellectual development and function						■					
	44	Consciousness											
	60	Recognizing											
	74	Psychomotor activity											
10	29	Temperament and personality									■		
	40	Performing an activity for an extended period (psychological endurance)								■			
	49	Expressing empathy		■									
	57	Affect										■	
	62	Managing general psychological demands										■	
	72	Energy and drive										■	
	88	Managing personal behaviour										■	
11	33	Managing a dangerous environment								■			
	90	Responding to dangers										■	

Concept mapping

For all 95 terms in the concept mapping we calculated the percentage of people who had problems with the term in the first eight questions for each item. Table 3 lists the items for which 25% or more of the respondents reported problems.

Table 3. Problematic items and dimensions: results of concept mapping in The Netherlands

Needs clarification
– Community (item and concept)
– Memory (concept)
– Thought, abstraction, judgement and related executive functions (item)
– Dressing appropriately (concept)
– Low vision/binocular (concept)

Difficult to use in the Dutch cultural context
– Community

Not useful for all age groups
– Community
– Economic self-sufficiency

Not useful for both genders: none

Not useful for all socioeconomic groups: none

Not useful for all ethnic/minority groups: none

Culturally sensitive (taboo)
– Experience of pain
– Keeping appropriate physical contact, and maintenance of social space
– Civic and community life
– Sexual functions
– Performing consensual sexual acts
– Incontinence

The Netherlands is a pluriform society, with an increasing percentage of people from different cultural and with different religious backgrounds. This makes it hard to indicate culturally sensitive items (question 8) for Dutch society as a whole. For instance, whereas The Netherlands is known to have rather liberal ideas about sexual matters there are some religious groups in Dutch society which take a puritan view of sexual functioning.

The Dutch respondents had many difficulties in indicating whether the different items referred to a function, to an activity or to participation (question 9). In no less than 72 of the 95 items more than 25% of the Dutch respondents indicated a level different to the levelé shown in the Beta-1 draft of ICIDH-2. For some items almost all respondents indicated the "wrong" level. Examples were "seeing" (item 3) and "interacting with an equal/co-worker/peer" (item 12).

On the basis of the results of question 10, on the importance of items, the 10 most important items according to the Dutch respondents are presented in Table 4. "Taking care of pets/domestic animals" (item 63), "cooking, baking and frying solids" (item 67) and "cultural activities" (item 52) were considered to be the most unimportant items.

Table 4. The 10 most important items: results of concept mapping in The Netherlands

1 and 2 *(equal):*
- Interpersonal and social relationships (item 31)
- Communication activities (item 55)

3–6 *(equal):*
- Taking care of one's health (item 28)
- Intellectual development and function (item 43)
- Affect (item 57)
- Managing personal behaviour (item 88)

7	Memory (item 4)
8	Language (item 81)
9	Managing close personal relationships (item 35)
10	Conversation processes and structure (item 68)

Focus groups

The medical professionals proposed nine areas of life activities, of which they considered three indispensable: self-care, social contacts with family and partner, and work/finances. Two more were under debate: well-being and dwelling (place to live). The six domains listed by WHO were prioritized as follows (from most to least important): self-care, getting on with people, life activities, moving and getting around, understanding and interacting with the world around you, and involvement in citizenship and economic life. The last two of these were considered dispensable if need be.

There were clear parallels between the categories proposed by the group and the WHO-provided domains considered indispensable. The domain of involvement in citizenship and economic life was considered abstract and difficult to understand and not vitally important, at least for chronic psychiatric patients. The impairments/activities mentioned for "Understanding and interacting with the world around you" were considered more a cause than a consequence of a health condition. It was felt that restrictions in this domain would automatically work through in the other domains, and thus the domain could be dispensed with.

Conclusion

The Dutch report on linguistic analysis comments on several problematic terms and some concern is expressed about the wording of some of the English annotations. The terms used in the measurement instrument must be in "plain" English to avoid trouble in translation. Careful rewording of some of the annotations is necessary to prevent misunderstandings caused not by the term itself but by the annotation attached. For a pluriform society it will be difficult to find terms that are not problematical for anybody. It is important to realize that translation problems may have influenced the results.

From the results of the concept mapping it is clear that the importance of the items varies. The type of respondent (e.g., patient, care-giver, professional) will probably influence views as to the importance of items. It might be advisable to compare the results for question 10 (the importance of the item within the framework) for all patients in the CAR study and the equivalent results for all care-givers. From the key informant interviews and self-administered questionnaire we learn that even highly educated people working at policy-making level have trouble in formulating "the view of society" on functioning and disablement. It may be less confusing to the respondent and yield more reliable data to focus on his/her personal view in future studies. Terminology involving a gradient (e.g., "quite mild") should be avoided or standardized. The format of the self-administered questionnaire was preferred to the format of the key informant interviews.

In The Netherlands, having good physical and mental health and functioning independently of others are positively valued. Personal freedom is also highly valued, and this extends to a climate of tolerance for "deviant" behaviour as long as it does not create a nuisance or danger for others. These aspects of society are reflected in the results of the CAR study in The Netherlands, and particularly the key informant interviews.

Chapter 13
Nigeria

O. Omigbodun, O. Odejide, and J. Morakinyo[*]

Highlights from the CAR study in Ibadan, Nigeria

- In Nigeria, strong negative attitudes towards persons with disabilities greatly limit their participation in society. Because of beliefs surrounding causation, this effect is more pronounced for persons with congenital and mental disabilities.

- There is a perceived urgent need for social assistance and other forms of aid to be provided for persons with disabilities as there is a general awareness of the absence of facilities to cater for the disabled.

- Existing legislation that may provide assistance for disabled workers applies only to government personnel.

- The national policy on education and the social development policy for Nigeria are two federal government policies with potential to help the disabled, but they have yet to be translated into binding laws.

- Public education about disabilities is urgently needed in our society. This could be used as an instrument for improving the lives of the disabled.

- ICIDH-2 will be useful for professionals and administrators for the assessment of disabilities, both for compensation purposes and for research activities.

Introduction

This centre report is based on data collected in the city of Ibadan, the capital of Oyo, one of the 36 states in Nigeria. Located in the south-west of Nigeria,

[*] Dept. of Psychiatry, College of Medicine, University of Ibadan, Nigeria.

Ibadan is inhabited predominantly by the Yoruba, one of the three main ethnic (language and culture) groups in Nigeria. It is home to the first university and teaching hospital in Nigeria as well as several research institutes and industries. As a result, there is a good mix of the local indigenous people and people from other ethnic groups who are attracted to the city by these institutions. To some extent, therefore, the results of the study reflect trends in other parts of Nigeria, since members of other ethnic groups who are resident in Ibadan were involved as respondents.

Nigeria's population is now estimated to be 116 million, with growth rate of 3% per annum. With a population of 4.1 million, Oyo is Nigeria's sixth most populous state. The population of the state is young, 44.9% are under the age of 15 years, 51.8% are aged between 15 and 64, and just 3.3% are aged over 65 (Federal Office of Statistics 1996).

Three pieces of existing legislation serve disabled workers: the *Workmen's Compensation Act* (1990); the *Nigerian Social Insurance Trust Fund* (1990); and the *Pensions Act* (1990). Unfortunately, this legislation applies only to government workers, leaving the rest of the population without support. The basis for compensation under these laws is limited to physical disabilities, leaving out the important section of the population suffering from mental disabilities. The laws involve paying workers financial compensation and pension benefits, without any provision for specific personal and social needs.

These are two additional federal government policies that may help the disabled, but they have yet to be translated into binding national laws. These are the National Policy on Education (1977; revised in 1981), which advocates the right to education for all citizens and the Social Development Policy for Nigeria (1989), which advocates the rehabilitation of all disabled persons. Both are important policy statements on federal goals, but neither has been given the necessary fiscal or infrastructure (systems) support to make them effective, apart from the backing they provide for nongovernmental organizations working on these issues.

Excerpt from Chapter 9 of Nigeria's Social Development Policy

"The fundamental objectives of the policy are to guarantee the total development of [the disabled persons'] human potentialities. It is particularly aimed at developing [their] capacity to meet the challenges of the disability and contemporary living, and ensure the attainment of a satisfactory overall quality of life which allows them to make their maximum contribution towards the development of the nation."

Whenever these policies are implemented, the quality of life of the disabled should change for the better and the burden of care should be greatly reduced for their blood relatives.

Methods

Instruments

The Nigerian site completed all components of the CAR study. These were: the international comparative analysis of legislation affecting the mental health aspects of impairments, disabilities and handicaps; key informant interviews, followed by the self-administered questionnaire; pile sort; concept mapping; translation and linguistic analysis; and focus group studies (Study 1: The Disablement Process Model and Study 2: Parity and Stigmatization of Disablements). An additional 10 concepts were included in the concept-mapping matrix by the Nigerian centre. These were: shaping and directing conversation, continence, working independently, handling own social position/social responsibilities, sexual interest, language, preparing food, taking decisions, having intimate relationships, and movement pattern in walking.

Sample

Fifteen subjects participated in the key informant interviews and self-administered questionnaire. The sample consisted of three medical professionals, three health policy-makers, one allied health professional, three physical health consumers/care-givers and five ADM health consumers or care-givers. The mean age of the key informant was 53.3 (SD=11.7), with a range of 26–76 years. Nine (60%) were female and six (40%) were male. Six reported having worked or were currently working in the area of physical disabilities, seven in mental health, and 4 in the alcohol and drug field.

A second sample (N=30) completed the concept mapping and pile sort instruments. Four subjects were medical professionals in the area of physical health, 10 were medical/allied health professionals in the area of ADM health, five were physical health consumers or care-givers, and 11 were ADM health consumers or care-givers. The mean age of the sample was 36.9 years (SD= 8.7). One of the female health professionals would not disclose her age. There were 19 males and 11 females. Thirteen reported having worked or were currently working in the physical disabilities area, 13 in the mental health area, and 13 in the alcohol/drug area. Five subjects reported ever having a physical disability, four reported ever having a mental disability, and one reported ever having an alcohol/drug problem.

Both samples were recruited between March and April 1997. Professionals were recruited using purposive sampling procedures. Potential subjects were visited either in their offices or at home, and the purpose of the study and its procedures were explained to them. The ADM and physical health consumers were recruited from NGO rehabilitation centres, hospital wards and outpatient clinics.

Procedures

All subjects had the option of coming to the site or being visited by an interviewer at their homes or in their offices. The scarcity of gasoline in the country during the period of study and the general lack of telephone facilities made transportation and communication rather difficult and expensive for the project.

Results

Key informant interviews and self-administered questionnaire

Qualitative analysis

Qualitative analysis of the interviews revealed that in Nigeria, the word "handicapped" is used to refer to activity limitation and lack of participation, and to a lesser extent to impairment. It serves as a partial cover term for disabled. The interviews also identified a number of derogatory terms such as "daft," "useless," "lazy," "imbecile" and "socially deficient" which are also used by the general public to refer to these concepts in ordinary conversations.

Key informants said that persons with disabilities would have great difficulty getting employment and getting married because of the significant level of bias against them in Nigerian society. This difficulty appeared to affect both physical and mental problems to a high degree. Persons with disabilities are seen as liabilities, and are viewed as people with low productivity in a society where survival is difficult for the non-disabled. However, they would find it easier to get married if they came from wealthy families who could afford to pay a big dowry and provide maintenance funds.

According to the key informants, disabilities that are present from birth, do not attract as much as sympathy as those caused by road traffic accidents.

This is because disabilities from birth are viewed as a curse or as a punishment for sin from God, while accidents are generally seen as something that could happen to anyone.

There was an extensive discussion among the key informants on the issue of social assistance from the government to the disabled, with a wide variation in responses. Despite being aware that disability services from the government are not readily available, the key informants had some difficulty in responding to this question. Their views generally reflected the range of attitudes in the society at large. However, they all considered that social assistance should be given when available, as long as the condition was not self-induced.

Quantitative analysis

Stigma ratings
Of the 18 health conditions presented, the three least stigmatizing conditions were being wheelchair-bound, being unable to read, and being blind. These were conditions that were not seen as being the fault of the person with the condition, and were conditions that deserved remediation. The three most stigmatizing conditions were leprosy, having a criminal record for burglary, and drug addiction.

Public reaction ratings
When the key informants were asked about the public reaction to the 10 conditions presented, the three that were thought to elicit the most negative reactions in Nigeria were being visibly under the influence of drugs, being visibly drunk, and being dirty and unkempt. The conditions eliciting the least negative reactions were: woman in the her 8th month of pregnancy, a person in a wheelchair, and an obese person.

Rank order of disability
Key informants were presented with the ranking cards and asked to rank disablements from the least to the most disabling. The three conditions perceived as the most disabling were two physical disabilities and one mental condition. These were, in rank order, quadriplegia, paraplegia, and active psychosis. The three least disabling conditions were, in mean rank order, vitiligo on the face, infertility, and total deafness.

Activities
Calculations of the average rating for the likelihood that people would be surprised if the person did certain activities, across all 10 activities, were

made for each of the five health conditions. Results revealed the following order of conditions, from least likely to most likely to elicit surprise:

- Persons born with low intelligence
- Persons with alcohol problems
- Persons in a wheel-chair
- Persons who hear voices
- Persons with heroin problems

The same calculation was done for the question "Is it likely that anyone would place restrictions or barriers on the person?" The order, from least likely to most likely to face barriers, was:

- Persons born with low intelligence
- Persons in a wheelchair
- Persons with alcohol problems
- Persons who hear voices
- Persons with heroin problems

The change in the position of alcohol problems in these two lists is an indication of the complexity of public response to problem drinking and alcohol addiction.

Concept mapping and pile sorting

The concept mapping exercise allowed respondents to identify problematic items in ICIDH-2, according to 10 dimensions of clarity, cultural sensitivity, comprehensibility, and usefulness to the classification.

Needs clarification
The items identified as posing problems of clarity included: mobility (item and definition), community (definition), and affect (item).

Difficult to use in culture
The items identified as culturally sensitive or posing some problem in usage were: use of communication devices; managing a dangerous environment; people sharing living space; communication content; performing consensual sexual acts; and sexual interest.

Not useful for all age groups

A number of items were identified as not being applicable to all age groups. These included: civic and community life; organizing daily routine; handling everyday physical environment; performing an activity for an extended period; self-care; work; people sharing living space; expressing empathy; problem solving; planning/organizing meals; cultural activities; handling technical devices/aids for locomotion; following events that take place outside of the direct environment; study behaviours; written communication; managing general psychological demands; taking care of pets/domestic animals; communication content; transferring oneself; interacting with an equal/co-worker/peer; recognizing direction in time and space; and keeping appropriate physical contact and maintenance of social space.

As can be seen by the length of the list, these items from ICIDH-2 were evaluated in terms of its orientation to primarily adult concerns. Many of the tasks listed would not be sensitive to children's issues because they are tasks that children would not be expected to perform, or tasks that they were not yet able to perform because of their stage of development, irrespective of their ultimate ability to perform them. The same is true of the applicability of the list to the elderly. Many of these tasks were seen as conditions that the elderly would not be expected to perform, or that were beyond their capacity to perform at their age. In effect, therefore, the list suggests that more attention needs to be given to the age consistency of the classification.

Culturally sensitive (taboo)

A number of items in the classification were recognized by the respondents as being important, but also being of a culturally sensitive nature. These included: dating and forming relationships; sexual functions; performing consensual sexual acts; sexual interest; and intimate relationships.

Discussion

The concepts of ICIDH-2

The concepts of impairment, activity limitation and lack of participation are yet to be clearly understood and accepted in the Nigerian culture. The results from the key informant interviews show that the concepts of impairment, activity limitation and lack of participation have yet to be fully understood and accepted in Nigerian culture. That culture considers disability as being synonymous with handicap and the aspect of participation is not yet fully appreciated. These differences in understanding are further buttressed by the definitions used in the blueprint on education of the handicapped in Nigeria (Federal Ministry of Education 1981). In this document, disability is defined as "a general term connoting physical, mental and social deviation from socially accepted norms which are medically confirmed" and handicap is defined as "a condition or an inability to perform certain functions because of a disability, e.g., reading, speaking, hearing." From these definitions it is obvious that the interpretation given by the policy-makers is quite different to that found in ICIDH-2.

Results of the pile sorting and concept mapping also reveal that several concepts were problematic on all dimensions, and most subjects had problems in rating items in the various concepts. These findings point to an unmet need for education. Policy-makers, professionals, persons with disabilities and their care-givers as well as the general populace would benefit from training sessions and public enlightenment campaigns to sensitize them to these concepts.

Negative attitudes towards persons with disabilities

Negative attitudes limit the participation of people with disabilities in society.

The society's negative perception of the disabled limits their participation in that society. The negative attitude is so strong that the differences in attitude towards the physically and the mentally disabled are sometimes blurred, or indistinguishable. While there is some evidence of a more negative perception of mental illness, the strength of the bias against all forms of disability make this a less critical issue for intervention at the present time than the overall treatment of all the disabled, combined.

These attitudes were further substantiated in the key informant interviews, where it was considered that the general populace believed that gaining employment, getting married and having a family would be severely affected. For mental illness, most informants commented that if problems started after marriage, the persons concerned would be sent packing and their children taken from them. However, the strong influence of wealth and support received from extended families in Nigerian society is exemplified by the view that persons with disabilities from wealthy families find it easier to get married.

Myths about causation

Myths about what causes disability have marked effects on societal attitudes towards persons with disabilities. The belief systems in the society surrounding causation of disabilities greatly influence the degree of sympathy received. Key informants stressed that society believes that congenital disabilities occur as a result of sin committed by the parents. The family and person affected are therefore viewed with great suspicion and lack of pity. This could even lead to such persons being abandoned by the family.

Mass education concerning the etiology of disabilities is urgently needed in our society. In a blueprint prepared by the Federal Ministry of Education (1981), it was remarked that the general feeling of the populace is that the handicapped are already "downtrodden and out," and that therefore any effort made to lift them up is money thrown down the drain.

Social assistance to the disabled

Social assistance from the Government is not clearly defined and there is a lack of parity between physical and mental health conditions. Nigeria's legislation on the care of the disabled is largely influenced by international conventions or treaties such as the English *Factories Act* of 1937 and the International Labour Organization (ILO) Health Services Conventions of 1985.

Existing legislation focuses on disabled workers. The policy is to provide them with either compensation or pension benefits. A medical board report is required to certify that the employee is incapable of working because of physical or mental illness. The federal or state government constitutes a medical board as and when necessary to review cases. In the private sector, a medical report from a physician is all that is required. There are no standardized procedures for assessment and the emphasis in the laws is more on physical than on mental problems.

Furthermore, the existing legislation is not sufficiently explicit regarding persons who have mental problems. For example, under the *Workmen's Compensation Act* "the claimant must be a worker under the act (sections 1 and 2) and must have suffered fatality (sections 3 and 4) or total incapacity permanently (section 5) or partial total incapacity (section 6) or temporary incapacity." The form of the incapacity is not further clarified in the Act.

Monetary compensation is determined according to the percentage of basic earnings lost per injury sustained. Virtually none of the statutory provisions expressly specify application to persons with mental disorders. The unavailability of social assistance to the disabled in the general populace was clearly indicated in the views of key informants. There was a wide variation in responses. Some believed that the government should provide assistance, while others felt that the person's relations should carry the burden. Still others considered that Nigerian society would never expect assistance to be given, no matter the duration of the illness.

The issue of causation was clearly reflected in the key informants' view that social assistance should never be accorded for substance abuse because it was self-induced. These opinions raise policy issues that need to be dealt with.

Several concepts not useful

Several of the disability concepts were not useful for all age groups and disabilities relating to sexual functions are seen as culturally sensitive in Nigeria. In the concept mapping exercise, a number of items were identified as not being useful for all age groups. This aspect needs further investigation. Was it due to a lack of understanding of the items? Furthermore, many of the items may not be applicable in the Nigerian culture. Activities relating to sexual functioning were identified as culturally sensitive, i.e., taboo. This finding is not surprising as in Nigerian society, such issues are not spoken about openly.

Conclusion

The involvement of the Ibadan centre in the project of the CAR study has been an enlightening experience for those involved. It has further stimulated health workers at the centre to focus more on the consequences of disabilities. The centre looks forward to disseminating the findings to policy-makers, health professionals, persons with disabilities and the society at large.

Chapter 14
Romania

*Radu Vrasti, Aurora Jianu, Ioan Drut, Marina Badoi,
and Hermine Iobb**

Highlights from the CAR study in Romania

- People with disabilities are supported by three national systems and protected by national law. Despite this, gaps remain and prejudice is prevalent.
- Romanian attitudes toward people with disabilities are frequently negative.
- Romanian words are able to capture the entire technical vocabulary used in the disablement phenomenon.
- The pile sorting results were consistent with the ICIDH-2 categories, suggesting cultural applicability of these dimensions of disability.
- Despite some confusion in terminology, the overall conceptual model is culturally appropriate and meaningful.

Introduction

Description of centre and regional area

This report is based on data collected in Timis district by the WHO Collaborating Centre and the Research Department of the 450-bed General Psychiatric Hospital at Jebel, which is the main psychiatric hospital in this part of Romania.

Jebel is a small town 24 km from Timisoara. Timis district has an area of 8,678 km^2 and a population of 700,292 (1991 national census). With a popu-

* Psychiatric Hospital, 1922 Jebel, Timis, Romania.

lation density of 80 per km². Timisoara, the capital of Timis district and Romania's second city, has about 350,000 inhabitants. According to the 1991 national census, 51.6% of the population of Timis district is female and 48.4% is male; 60.7% of the population lives in urban areas. Timis district is the catchment area for the Jebel Psychiatric Hospital, which has about 3000 admissions each year. The clientele of the hospital spans virtually all categories of mental health patients (chronic and acute, psychotic and psychopathic disorders, patients with mental retardation, alcohol and drug dependence, etc.).

Romanian support system for disabilities

The Romanian disability support system encompasses three schemes:

1. The pension for invalidity scheme (pension for medical reasons), financed by workplace taxes and provided by the Ministry of Labour, which assures income for individuals who have undergone a temporary (at least 6 months) or permanent restriction of work performance due to physical illness, injuries, mental disorders, or alcohol and drug problems. This scheme uses a three-dimension classification according to work performance and functioning in everyday life (i.e., whether domestic support is needed).

2. The benefit for handicapped people scheme, financed by the State Secretariat for Handicapped People, provides an income, special protection and other benefits for people who qualify as handicapped. This scheme is based on whether an assistant is needed to manage in everyday life.

3. The social assistance (welfare) scheme provided by the Ministry of Labour to persons who are unable to be self-supporting and to manage in daily life (mostly homeless people or those with mental retardation).

Brief analysis of national policy for the protection of disabled people

According to the *Law about Special Protection of Handicapped People* (1992): "... handicapped people are those individuals who, because of sensorial, physical or mental deficiencies, are not able to integrate, partially or totally, temporarily or permanently, through their own capacities, in social and professional life, and require special protection."

The State Secretariat for Handicapped People is a national agency dedicated to the protection, education and rehabilitation of people with handicaps. A subsidiary organ of the State Secretariat, the so-called Territorial

State Inspectorate for Handicapped People, is present in each district. This department is responsible for the assessment and certification of disabled people as people with handicaps who are authorized to receive handicapped persons' benefits under the national regulations.

According to the severity of impairment of work performance, handicapped people are divided into three categories: the first encompasses handicapped individuals who need an assistant for everyday life, the second contains people whose life is very restricted because of their medical diagnosis, and the third covers people who are only partially restricted in their activities.

Traditional views of disability in Romanian culture

There are two ways of defining and referring to disabilities in Romania: one describes disabled people in terms of illness and abnormality, and the other depicts them as unhappy people who have been punished for their faults, or as unlucky.

Romanian people have a negative attitude towards people with disabilities and health professionals have demonstrated similar views. In the lay vocabulary, many pejorative words and expressions that convey a fatalistic perception of the destiny of persons with disabilities are used. In brief, Romanians view health as a virtue and disability as a sin.

Methods

Procedures

The Jebel Collaborating Centre completed all components of the CAR study.

Sample

Pile sorting

Thirty subjects were recruited for the pile sorting exercise, drawn from groups:
- 10 subjects working in the area of mental disabilities (health professionals): mean age 39.0±9.7 years (range 28–57); 1 male: 9 females; education: 17.7±3.16 years of schooling; 7 psychiatrists and psychologists, 2 nurses, and 1 other health worker.

- 10 subjects with mental disabilities or alcohol and drug problems or their care-givers: mean age 40.9±7.44 (range 23–48); 2 males; 8 females; education; 14.7±3.36 years of schooling.

- 5 subjects working in the area of physical disabilities (health professionals): mean age 41.2±9.03 years; 5 males: no females; education, 19.6±3.04 years of schooling.

- 5 subjects with physical disabilities or their care-givers: mean age 38.0±7.71years; 2 males; 2 females; education: 12.2±8.36 years of schooling.

Key informant interview and self-administered questionnaire

Fifteen subjects participated in the key informant interviews: 3 persons with disabilities; 3 care-givers; 3 medical professionals; 3 disability specialists and 3 policy-makers or opinion leaders. The mean age of the key informant was 43.8±7.48 years (range 33–57); there were nine males and six females, with an average of 16.2±2.60 years of schooling.

Concept mapping

Thirty subjects completed the concept mapping exercise – 24 from the pile sorting contained 10 medical professionals in the area of alcohol, drug and mental (ADM) disorders, 10 ADM health consumers or their care-givers, five medical professionals in the area of physical health, and five physical health consumers or their care-givers. The mean age of the sample was 40.6±8.64 years (range 24–57); these were 17 males and 13 females.

Focus group

In accordance with the overall study design, the Jebel Collaborating Centre performed two focus group studies: one exploring the underlying model of the ICIDH-2 classification and another exploring the stigma attached to disabilities in Romanian culture. For each study, we used two groups: eight health professionals currently working with disabled people (mean age 44.2±4.97 years, three men and five women, and seven disabled individuals (mean age 46.5±4.07 years, three men and four women).

Results

Linguistic analysis

Romanian words were able to capture the full meaning of the technical vocabulary used to encompass the disability phenomenon. The most difficult problem was to distinguish between "illness," "disease," and "sickness." In the Romanian language, all three words are synonymous, having the same core meaning and connotations. Finding an equivalent for "impairment" was another problem, because the main meaning of the most appropriate Romanian word – *afectare* (affectation) – is much more closely related to damage, deterioration, spoil age or breakage than to loss of body function. For the English word, "handicap," there is a similar Romanian word, *handicap,* but its meaning in relation to disabled people is very new. Its commonest use is as a sports term.

Pile sorting study

Each subject who completed the pile sorting exercise selected on average 10.0±2.74 piles (range 6–18 piles). Analysing the complete sample, we found that seven pile groups were chosen most frequently. Their title can be roughly translated into the following: cognition, communication, mobility, sensation, domestic activities, work, and basic functions.

It was noted that health professionals working in the ADM disabilities domain produced more piles than disabled people or care-givers. Activities encompassed in the various piles generally corresponded to clusters that are included in the ICIDH-2 classification of impairments, activities, and participation. In this sense, the results suggest that these dimensions are cross-culturally applicable, at least with regard to Romania.

Key informant interview and self-administered questionnaire

Terms and concepts for disabilities used in Romanian culture

- For "impairment," a majority of respondents said that "the majority of people living here" used such words as "ill," "infirm" or "impotence."
- For "disability," the majority of our informants mentioned "incapable," "inapt" or even "handicapped." The general meaning is related to func-

tioning, but there is also a confusion (overlapping) between loss of function and handicap.

- With regard to social participation; most respondents chose the word "handicapped," though a minority chose "invalid." In sum, to be unable to do something means to be a handicapped person.

In general, "impairments" were referred to in terms demoting illness and "disabilities" in terms of functioning. For the majority of people, "disability" and "handicap" were labels that referred to a loss of function or body part.

Threshold of public perception of disability

- Concerning people with mobility problems, almost all informants focused on physical signs for noticing a problem, seeing it as serious, or viewing the person as needing help (for attention: *difficulty walking, avoid walking;* for seriousness: *need support, falling down;* for needing help: *difficulties in food provision, in walking, sustaining body position*).
- People with mental disorders were noticed by the community because of their disturbed behaviour or bizarre ideas.
- People with low intelligence were thought to be recognizable by language and communication disorders and childish behaviour, and an inability to care for themselves.
- People with alcohol problems were thought to be recognizable because they neglected their obligations, behaved irritably, and prompted family conflicts and problems at work. People with drug problems were thought to show bizarre and changed behaviour or antisocial behaviour.
- In general, there was only a small difference between the thresholds of noticing a problem and viewing it as serious.

Rank-order of disabilities

In the rank-ordering exercise, the five most disabling conditions were considered to be quadriplegia, dementia, active psychosis, paraplegia, and total blindness.

Social stigma

The five least stigmatized conditions were blindness, depression, being wheelchair- bound, obesity, and inability to read. Conversely, the most stigmatizing conditions were criminal records for burglary, drug addiction, and homelessness.

Public reaction

Participants thought that the public would view people under the influence of drugs or alcohol, people with a chronic mental disorder, or those who were dirty and unkempt the most negatively.

Focus group

Both health professionals and individuals with disabilities were able to distinguish between the concepts of impairment and disability, but the meanings and definitions differed somewhat between groups. Health professionals viewed impairment as "static" and at the body level, and disability as "dynamic" and at the level of overall functioning. People with ADM disabilities viewed impairment as an affliction of body structure and disability as a restriction of function. For both groups, it was more difficult to make the distinction between disability and handicap, as both terms have the same meaning in lay vocabulary. As a whole, though, the health professionals better captured the ICIDH-2 definitions.

The overall model of disability was understandable for health professionals and was considered to be helpful to them in their normal work. The people with disabilities had some difficulties with the terminology and meaning of societal participation. In general, the model appears adequate for health professionals working with disabled people, but it is not as appropriate for people with disabilities or health and social agencies.

Most focus group participants felt that Romanian attitudes toward people with disabilities are frequently negative. Negative attitudes are often expressed in terms of exclusion from various aspects of life such as relationships, employment and access to community facilities. People with ADM disabilities were thought to experience greater levels of rejection than those with physical disabilities. Rural communities were thought to be more tolerant than those in urban areas. People with little education were seen as intolerant towards those with ADM disabilities but relatively more tolerant and supportive towards physically disable individuals.

As a reflection of the negative attitude towards disabled persons, it was noted that Romanian people use many pejorative words to describe those with disabilities.

On a more positive note, focus group participants noted the recent implementation of laws and regulations concerning assistance for people with disabilities, including financial support, the use of care-givers, encouragement to hire disabled people in the workplace, and the development of nongovernmental associations supporting handicapped people.

Conclusion

In Romania, the general public has a negative attitude towards disabled people. This is particularly true in the case of mental-drug- or alcohol-related disabilities. Some recent progress has been made, however, including new laws and the provision of financial support. Despite some confusion regarding terminology, the overall conceptual model of disability in ICIDH-2 is culturally appropriate and meaningful.

Chapter 15
Spain

*J.L. Vázquez-Barquero, S. Herrera Castanedo, M. Uriarte Ituiño,
I. Lastra Martinez, and E. Vázquez Bourgón**

Highlights from the CAR study in Spain

* Spain has progressed politically towards a federal system, in which the 17 different regions or autonomous communities are increasingly able to shape their own health and social security systems.

* The basic national provision for disability support in Spain is part of the general health system, which provides payment for sick leave from work. For severe disabilities that limit the ability to work, there is a social security system providing sick benefits and a pension.

* The first law to regulate aspects related to disabilities and handicaps in Spain was the LISMI (*Social Integration Law for Handicapped People*, 1982). The main goal of this law is to prevent discrimination against persons with physical or mental disabilities.

* However, parity does not exist between physical and mental health conditions in some respects, for instance disability benefits and work opportunities.

* The degree of social disapproval in Spain is linked more to people's attitudes, stereotypes, and cultural opinions than to illness.

Introduction

In recent years, Spain has progressed politically towards a federal system, in which the 17 different regions or autonomous communities are increasingly able to shape their own health and social security systems.

* Unidad de Investigacion en Psiquiatria Clinica y Social, Santander, Spain.

Thus, progressively we are able to detect regional variations in extension of the coverage for disabilities, which depends on the political interest of the different political parties governing each region. In general Spain has a welfare system covering 100% of the population. State welfare covers the following aspects:

- All health conditions. Acute or chronic diseases are covered. In certain conditions – e.g., mental illness – there are also additional services developed by local authorities. Rehabilitation and prevention programmes for disabilities are, however, not fully developed in all regions.

- Social security system. This system is divided into two basic levels: *contribution level*, directed to all workers who have paid the social security taxes during their employment period; and no *contribution level*, directed to people who have never reached the minimum salary established by law.

The first law to regulate aspects of disabilities and handicaps in Spain was the LISMI (*Social Integration Law for Handicapped People, 1982*). The main goal of this law is to prevent discrimination against persons with physical or mental disabilities. There are also regulations to stimulate industries to employ disabled persons. In addition to the national disability support structure, there are some powerful nongovernmental organizations which cover specific disabilities.

Family support is still very strong in Spanish society. This is reflected, for example, in the fact that a high proportion of persons with disabilities or mental illness live with their families.

Our region, Cantabria, is an autonomic community with an area of 5298 km² situated in the northern coastal part of Spain. It has a population of nearly 600,000 inhabitants. The area and the population represent 1.05% and 1.27%, respectively, of the national totals. The active population (200,200 inhabitants) is divided almost equally into three sectors: (i) agriculture, mainly dairy farming; (ii) industry; and (iii) commerce and services. Cantabria does not have different ethnic groups, and the majority of the population belongs to the Roman Catholic religion.

Methods

For the CAR project, our unit established links with different organizations working in the field of disabilities in Cantabria. All data were gathered in the region of Cantabria between February and May 1997.

Instruments and procedures

The Spanish site completed all basic components of the CAR study: centre description, linguistic analysis, key informant interviews, pile sorting, concept mapping, and focus group interviews.

Sample

Pile sorting and concept mapping

A total of 30 individuals were selected to complete both exercises, divided into two broad categories:

- Medical and other health professionals ($N=15$)
- Consumers and care-givers ($N=15$)

The mean age of this sample was 39.4 (SD=11.6). Thirteen (43%) subjects were female, and 17 (57%) were male. Of the 15 professionals, seven reported ever working in the physical disabilities area, 14 in the mental health area, and nine in the alcohol/drug area. Only two subjects reported ever having a physical disability, four reported ever having a mental disability; and seven reported having an alcohol/drug problems.

Key informants in Cantabria

The sample for this exercise (18 people) was divided into six groups: three persons with physical disabilities, three persons with mental disabilities, three medical professionals, three mental health professionals, three social workers, care-givers, therapists, and three policy makers or opinion leaders in the area of disability services. The mean age of this group was 41.6 (SD=13.38). Ten (55.6%) subjects were female, and eight (44.4%) were male. Four people reported ever working in the area of physical disabilities, nine reported ever working in the area of mental health; and 7 ever worked in the alcohol/ drug field.

Focus groups

In total, there were two focus groups. The first group comprised 12 people, including six individuals with disability and six family members of disabled people. The second group included 11 health professionals from various professional specialities.

Results

Linguistic analysis

Analysis of the 44 items included in list A

The majority of the items were easily transferable to Spanish, and we obtained a 61.3% equivalency between the original terms in English and the resulting terms after the back-translation process. However, there are some problematic concepts. We used the linguistic evaluation protocol to analyse the nature of these problems.

1. Concepts that were difficult to translate because there is no exact equivalent term in Spanish.
   Original term: Disablement
   Translation into Spanish: *Minusvalidez*
   Back-translation: Handicap

   The term "disablement" is intended to cover all domains related to impairment, disability and participation, and is used as an umbrella term to describe the process. In Spanish no equivalent term exists and the closest term does not describe the disability process.

2. The term in Spanish has a narrower meaning than the original term.
   Original term: Health condition
   Translation into Spanish: *Estado de salud*
   Back-translation: State of health

   The term in Spanish does not include some of the conditions that lead to a contact with a health agency, such as "pregnancy."

3. The term in Spanish has a broader than found in the original.
   Original term: Handling everyday physical environment
   Translation into Spanish: *Autonomía física*
   Back-translation: Physical autonomy

4. Two or more items from the ICIDH-2 translate into the same term in Spanish, and the distinctions between the original items are lost.
   Original term: Disease
   Translation into Spanish: *Enfermedad*
   Back-translation: Illness, disease

In Spanish the terms "illness" and "disease" are equivalent and translated as "*enfermedad.*"

Analysis of the 67 items included in list B

It is difficult to determine the percentage of equivalency for this list because it consists of long sentences, but generally speaking we consider that an adequate conceptual equivalence was achieved.

Key informant interviews and self-administered questionnaire

The qualitative analysis of section A of the questionnaire revealed that in Spanish the words "disability" and "handicap" overlap, and that they are used interchangeably in the professional argot. There was more variability among patients, who showed no agreement about general terms meaning "activity limitation" and "participation restriction."

Regarding the person's ability to obtain a job, key informants said that there are few opportunities for persons with physical problems and none for persons with mental problems. All the informants said that it is very difficult for people with alcohol/drugs problems to find a job, and if they finally get one it would be even more difficult to keep it.

The majority of respondents said that the ability to get married and have a family would be affected if the person has a mental, alcohol or drug problem but they did not see it as a general problem if the person has a physical disability. There was agreement among informants that social assistance from the government should be immediate for people who are unable to work as a consequence of a physical or mental problem. Opinions were divided whether social assistance should be available for people with an alcohol or drug problem.

We decided to create a database file for the rank-order task on relative disability in order to facilitate the data analysis and interpretation. Using the SPSS Program, we entered data related to case number (1–18), type of informant and the 17 variables that were ranked by the participants. Once all data were entered, we applied descriptive statistical methods. With the data we were able to show the hierarchical structure of disabilities. Calculating the mean score for each variable related to a heath condition and assuming that the one with the highest score was considered the least disabling and the one with the lowest was the most disabling, we developed the rank-order scores in Table 1.

Table 1. Rank order of health conditions by severity

Health condition	Rank	Mean	Deviation	Median	N
Quadriplegia	1	2.61	3.09	2.00	18
Dementia	2	2.89	2.17	2.00	18
Depression	3	5.61	3.07	5.00	18
Paraplegia	4	6.00	3.31	5.50	18
Active psychosis	5	6.39	4.43	5.00	18
Total blindness	6	7.44	3.76	7.50	18
Alcoholism	7	8.28	2.61	8.50	18
Drug addiction	7	8.28	3.69	8.50	18
Total deafness	9	8.89	3.01	9.00	18
Mild mental retardation	10	9.28	2.67	10.00	18
HIV positive	11	10.83	4.71	12.50	18
Incontinence	12	11.72	3.86	12.00	18
Amputation	13	11.78	2.29	11.50	18
Migraines	14	11.83	3.38	13.00	18
Rheumatoid arthritis	15	12.06	3.30	14.00	18
Infertility	16	15.17	4.06	16.50	18
Vitiligo on face	17	15.2	3.38	16.00	18

Table 2. Ranking of degree of social disapproval

Health condition	Rank	Mean	Deviation	Median	N
Blindness	1	1.00	.39	1.00	16
Wheelchair bound	2	1.06	1.12	1.00	16
Depression	3	1.44	1.41	1.00	16
Inability to read	4	1.50	1.21	1.00	16
Borderline intelligence	5	2.56	1.31	2.00	16
Dementia	6	2.75	2.65	2.00	16
Obese	7	3.25	3.28	2.00	16
Facial disfigurement	8	4.88	2.83	5.00	16
Homeless	9	5.56	3.20	7.00	16
Chronic mental disorder	9	5.56	2.58	5.50	16
Someone who cannot hold a job	11	6.06	2.35	6.50	16
Alcoholism	12	6.63	2.00	7.00	16
Dirty and unkempt	13	7.00	1.93	7.00	16
Leprosy	14	7.19	2.61	8.00	16
Someone who cannot take care of their children	15	7.88	1.71	8.00	16
Criminal record for burglary	16	8.13	1.31	8.00	16
HIV positive	17	8.56	1.46	9.00	16
Drug addiction	18	8.69	1.66	9.00	16

Table 3. Social reaction to appearance in public

	People would think there was no issue, and would pay no attention	People would notice, but would not think there was any issue	People would be uneasy about it would probalby not do anything	People would be uneasy about it and try to avoid the person	People would think, it was wrong, and might say somthing about	People would think it was wrong, and would try to stop it
Someone with a chronic mental disorder who "acts out"		11.1%	11.1%	55.6% ✓	22.2%	
A woman in her eighth month of pregnancy	55.6% ✓	44.4%				
A person in a wheelchair	44.4%	55.6% ✓				
A person who is intellectually "slow"	16.7%	66.7% ✓	16.7%			
Someone who is dirty and unkempt		5.6%	27.8%	50% ✓	6.7%	
Someone with a face disfigured from burns	11.1%	22.2%	55.6% ✓	11.1%	16.7%	
An obese person	38.9%	44.4% ✓			16.7%	
Someone who is visibly drunk			11.1%	38.9%	44.4% ✓	5.56%
Someone who is visibly under the influence of drugs			5.6%	38.9%	55.6% ✓	
Someone who is blind	11.1% 83.3% a	5.6%				

The figures show the percentage of participants that ranked the box; ✓ indicates highest percentage for each condition

We also created a database file using the same statistical program for the task related to degree of social disapproval. We entered the case case number (1–18), the type of informant, and the 18 variables ranked by the informants scoring the degree of disapproval. Using all the data collected, and calculating the median score for each item on the list, we generated the hierarchical structure of the items, from the lowest degree of social disapproval to the highest, for our sample (see Table 2).

Following the same process, we created a data file containing information related to the social reaction task. In this case all the variables were categorical, so that statistical management of the results were different. Using a simple descriptive statistical method, we were able to delineate the global patterns of social reaction in our culture (see Table 3).

Concept mapping

Almost all the participants in this exercise found it long and irritating, and many mentioned that there were too many items. Many of the respondents started to answer the questions mechanically after the first 20 items, and we presume that this was the reason we did not obtain all the information expected from this exercise.

The concept mapping analysis yielded a list of items that were problematic for any of the 10 questions asked. Table 4 includes all the items for which 25% or more of the respondents reported problems.

Table 4. Problematic items for more than 25% of participants

Items	Type of problem
Mobility	Definition
Visual sensory functions	Item
Following written instructions	Definition
Managing general psychological demands	Item
Psychomotor activity	Item
Handling body-attached technical aids	Item
Keeping rules/abiding by decisions	Item
Sexual functions	Culturally sensitive (taboo)
Thought, abstraction, judgement and related executive functions	Item Definition Not useful for all socio-economic groups
Work acquisition and retention behaviours	Definition
Performing consensual sexual acts	Culturally sensitive (taboo)

Pile sorting

The raw data for each participant were typed as an ASCII file and imported into the computer program, ANTHROPAC 3.0, which has a data conversion routine that transforms raw pile sort data into an item-by-item similarities matrix. The matrix was analysed using multivariate statistics. This analysis revealed those items which associate more strongly and hence were more stable in our sample. At the same time, it showed items that were not included in any cluster and those with only very marginal association with the clusters.

The cut-point used as our reference was 0.3936, yielding 11 clusters (see Table 5). An "*" marks the items in the cluster that formed the strongest central tendency in the cluster; these are the most stable items in each cluster. By looking at these central items we can give a generic name or title to the clusters to identify the corresponding domains. The symbol "^" is used to represent the item or items in each cluster that were least strongly associated with the other items. These are items that either were associated with multiple clusters during the pile sort process, or were sometimes seen as isolates or difficult to classify with the other items.

Table 5. Pile sort exercise: distribution of items by cluster

Cluster N°	Domain's Name	Cluster composition
Cluster 1	Mobility	74^, 6, 38, 45, 1*, 56*, 66, 53, 75
Cluster 2	Sensory functions	11^, 19, 25, 3*, 26*.72^, 77^
Cluster 3	Affectivity	49*, 54*, 57
Cluster 4	Cognition and general abilities	40, 62, 21, 41, 29, 44, 13, 60, 9, 5, 4*, 7*, 43, 34, 69
Cluster 5	Training	59, 80
Cluster 6	Social and civic abilities	2, 22, 39, 12, 14, 47, 31, 23, 35*, 37*, 71, 76^, 83
Cluster 7	Communication	81^, 16^, 8, 18, 20, 55*, 64*
Cluster 8	Leisure activities	58, 15*, 52*, 73
Cluster 9	Daily life activities	36^, 28, 63, 24, 67, 51*, 70*, 10, 42, 30, 78, 84, 27, 32, 86, 87
Cluster 10	Economy and work	50^, 17, 65, 46, 82, 89^
Cluster 11	Self-protection	88^, 33*, 90*

Key: * = most stable items; ^ = least strongly associated items.

Focus group

The group containing individuals with disabilities and family members agreed with the importance of most domains of functioning set out in the ICIDH-2. However, they did not think that the domain "participation in society" was as relevant as the others. The health professional group, on the other hand, thought that this domain was important. They noted some overlap with the other five domains but agreed on the importance of these content areas.

General overview of CAR results

Table 6 provides a summary of all items that were problematic during performance of any exercise in the CAR study. This table is the result of combining the quantitative and qualitative findings of the linguistic analysis, pile sort and concept mapping exercises.

Table 6. Summary of all problematic items in the CAR study

Items	Type of problem	Exercise
Mobility	Concept	Concept mapping
Visual sensory functions	Item	Concept mapping
Following written instructions	Item	Concept mapping
Handling general psychological demands	Item Translation	Concept mapping Linguistic analysis
Psychomotor activity	Item Not stable in our culture	Concept mapping Pile sorting
Handling body-attached technical aids	Item Translation	Concept mapping Linguistic analysis
Keeping rules/abiding by decisions	Item Translation	Concept mapping Linguistic analysis
Sexual functions	Culturally sensitive (taboo) Not stable in our culture	Concept mapping Pile sorting
Performing consensual sexual acts	Culturally sensitive (taboo) Not stable in our culture Translation	Concept mapping Pile sorting Linguistic analysis
Though, abstraction, judgement and related executive functions	Item Concept Not valid for all socio-economic groups	Concept mapping
Work acquisition and retention behaviours	Item Translation	Concept mapping Linguistic analysis
Language	Not stable in our culture	Pile sorting

Table 6 (continued)

Managing personal behaviour	Not stable in our culture Translation	Pile sorting Linguistic analysis
Energy and drive	Not stable in our culture Translation	Pile sorting Linguistic analysis
Responding to conversational cues	Not stable in our culture	Pile sorting
Following (showing interest in) events that take place outside the direct environment	Not stable in our culture	Pile sorting
Problem-solving	Not stable in our culture	Pile sorting
Handling everyday physical environment	Translation	Linguistic analysis
Using of special means of communication	Translation	Linguistic analysis
Use of communication devices	Translation	Linguistic analysis
Managing dangerous environment	Translation	Linguistic analysis
Monitoring and evaluating of performance of activities/tasks	Translation	Linguistic analysis

Conclusion

The CAR project, apart from offering reliable information about the cross-cultural applicability of the ICIDH-2, provided an excellent opportunity to give feedback on the conceptual structure, linguistic style and use of English terms in the classificatory system. As a result of this information we were able to report some conclusions derived from each part of the project.

Regarding the results obtained in the linguistic analysis, we can conclude that items used in the ICIDH-2, are easily transferable to our language. The 61.3% equivalency for list A and analysis of list B indicate that we can develop a conceptually adequate translation of the ICIDH-2 in Spanish.

The key informants results revealed that the terms "disability and handicap" are used interchangeably in Spanish, and the boundaries between them are not clear in our culture. Section B indicated that in Spain alcohol and drug addiction are not seen so much as illnesses but as behaviours. Alcohol problems are better tolerated than drug addiction in our society. People with these sorts of problems are seen as being responsible for them, which affects in a determinant way the social assistance they should get from the system. In general, physical disabilities are better understood and regarded than mental disabilities in our country. It is important to note, the high ranking given to depression in Table 1, which leads us to think that our society is improving a great deal in its understanding the consequences of this mental disorder.

The results of the concept mapping clearly indicate the items that were problematic in our culture. Those items should be noted in the revision process, since more than 25% of participants in the task thought that they were not clear enough to be retained in the classification, and need to be defined or worded in some other way. Only two items (sexual functions and performing consensual sexual acts) were culturally sensitive, indicating that in our society, matters regarding sexual relationships are taboo or difficult to talk about.

The cluster analysis of the pile sort data revealed that there some of the concepts are confusing and unstable in our culture. This analysis also suggested that there are differences between professionals and patients. The revision of these items should be directed to finding out the reasons that made them confusing.

Chapter 16
Tunisia

Adel Chaker*

Highlights from the CAR Study in Tunisia

- In Tunisia, disability associated with mental and alcohol- or drug-related disorders is discriminated against much more than disability due to physical disorders.
- If people are holders of an official "disability card," they receive an allowance even though they may already be the beneficiaries of the social security system and/or insurance schemes in the country.
- This official "disability card" may be obtained by meeting health criteria which are not well defined, and, as such, objectionable. Substance abuse is not included at all, and mental disability is defined solely as an intellectual deficiency.
- Access to specialized assistance such as specialized education, rehabilitation and professional training, can be obtained only through the use of the "disability card."
- Despite some problems with terminology and the applicability of concepts to all societal sectors, the overall ICIDH-2 conceptual model of disability is culturally appropriate and meaningful in Tunisia.

Introduction

Tunisia is a southern Mediterranean country located in North Africa between the western and eastern drainage basins of the Mediterranean Sea. This area is 155,566 km², and Islam is the State religion. Tunisia has 23 governovates. The CAR study was conducted in the 3 governovates, of Tunis, the capital

* Centre d'Appareillage, Orthopédique, Manouba, Tunisia.

city, Ariana and Ben Arous. According to the most recent census (1994), the population of Tunisia is 8,815,400. Of these, 5.4% are aged 65 years or older, 59.8% are aged 15–64, and 34.8% are aged under 15 years. The population of Tunis itself is 1,836,800 (20.8 % of the population of the country. (National Institute of Statistics, 1994)

Being disabled in Tunisia

Statistical data on disability

In Tunisia, the censuses carried out in 1975, 1984, and 1994 by the National Institute of Statistics are the principal sources of statistical information on persons with disabilities in the country. A national survey on employment (EPE 89) was also undertaken by the National Institute of Statistics in 1989, and it is also a valuable source of statistical information in this field.

These two sources provide data on the prevalence of disability in the country as well as useful indications on sociodemographic characteristics at the national level (age, sex, type of housing, income-generating activities).

Table 1. Persons suffering from severe functional disabilities

	1975 census Population	Prevalence	1984 census P. I.		EPE 89 survey P. I.		1994 census P. I.	
Blind	12,400	0.221	12,110	0.174	9,300	0.117	16,931	0.2
Deaf or dumb	4,930	0.087	8,630	0.123	11,000	0.14	15,481	0.18
With sensory-motor impairments	12,360	0.221	21,890	0.313	17,000	0.215	43,710	0.5
Mentally retarded	7,000	0.125	14,070	0.202	13,100	0.166	29,078	0.33
Others	7,000	0.125	3,860	0.056	3,100	0.04	2,082	0.02
Total	43,700	0.782	60,500	0.87	53,500	0.676	107,282	1.2

The EPE 89 survey included data on disabilities that do not entail a drastic reduction in functional activities in the society, for example mild mental retardation, near-sightedness, paralysis induring no major hindrance for the individual, and other similar cases.

The number of these less severe cases was 41,600. Taking this into account the total number of all disabled people (mild cases and severe cases) is 95,500 or more than 1% of the population.

Definition of disability in Tunisian law

Tunisian law defines disability as a limitation of functional activities in the society for the individual, as specified in Law No. 81/46, 1981, which reads: "A person who is disabled experiences limitations in one or many key activities of daily life. These limitations include sensory, mental or motor functions of the individual." The great asset of this particular law is that it takes into account the key activities of daily life. At the same time, it has the weakness that the spectrum of possible causes of disability is not wide enough. Substance abuse (drugs and alcohol), for example, is not listed among possible causes of disability. Substance abuse can be included among the list of acquired causes of disability if sensory-motor functions of the body are impaired by those substances (e.g., neuritis or polyneuritis caused by alcohol dependence).

At present, the Tunisian social welfare system provides disabled persons with allowances, mainly social and financial help and compensation for injury at work or occupational disease.

The compensation scheme benefits only those who already contribute to the social security system (workers in general, interns, students, household help persons, prisoners, inpatients in mental health institutions, volunteers).

Procedures

The following six components were completed within the framework of the CAR study: Centre description questionnaire (results presented in introduction); translation and linguistic analysis; key informant interviews; concept mapping matrix; pile sorting; and focus group discussions.

Sampling

Key informant interviews

Fifteen people participated, including three specialists, three trainers, three administrators, three physicians, and three people with motor-related disabilities. Their average age was 35.8 years (± 5.9 years), 53.4% were male and 46.6% were female. The group was experienced in working with various types of impairments. Ten participants had worked with people who have motor impairments; 11 participants had experience with people who have mental impairments; and five had worked with people who have substance abuse-related problems.

Concept mapping matrix and pile sorting

Thirty people participated in this portion of the CAR study. The group included five physicians with experience in the field of physical handicap, 10 physicians with experience in the field of mental handicap, five people with motor impairments, and 10 people with mental impairments or alcohol-related problems. Collectively, their average age was 34.7 years (± 7.9 years); 15% were male and 15% were female.

Focus group

Two focus groups were conducted. The first group was composed of people with disabilities and their families. Six participants had physical impairments and four participants were family members (total $N=10$). The second group was comprised of health professionals in the disability field (total $N=8$): three physicians, one psychologist, two educators, one sociologist, and one administrator.

Results

Qualitative linguistic analysis

Words were found in the Arabic language that generally reflected the English disability terminology in the draft ICIDH-2.

In Arabic, the word "*iaka*" – handicap – is either (a) the reflection of a certain uncleanness, or (b) a more generic term expressing a functional disability/deficiency/flaw. "*Iaka*" can be used for people and/or objects and structures (such as a corporation for example).

In Arabic, the word "*ajz*" – incapacity – means deficiency in itself viewed from a purely functional angle, i.e., a certain task/function that cannot be achieved.

"*Iaka*" and "*ajz*" also can be interpreted as a restriction and/or limitation affecting the activities of individuals in society.

Key informant interview

Key informants felt that people suffering from motor impairments stand a better chance of finding a job or getting married and having a family than those with mental impairments or alcohol- or drug-related problems.

Informants also believed that stigma in society particularly affects those who abuse substances or have some sort of mental problem, whether acquired or hereditary. As a result, these people do not get much help from others because their disability is regarded with disdain, and because they are seen as sometimes complicating matters through their own behaviour.

Quantitative analysis

Stigma
Among all the 18 health conditions associated with stigma, those found to be least stigmatizing were obesity, using a wheelchair, and blindness. The most stigmatizing conditions were thought to be substance abuse, abandoning one's own children, and being HIV-infected.

Society and its reactions
Among the 10 health conditions proposed as stigmatizing *vis-à-vis* society, being unclean, being drunk, and being under the influence of drugs were thought to trigger very negative reactions from others. Conversely, being in a wheelchair, being blind, and being obese usually were judged to prompt the least negative reactions on the part of society.

Ranking exercise
Among all 17 health conditions listed as disabilities for this exercise, the following were considered most serious: being HIV-infected, being quadriplegic, and suffering from dementia. Conditions viewed as least serious were rheumatism, vitiligo, and migraine.

Cultural barriers and acceptance
Among the five scenarios describing individuals with disabilities, and among the 10 tasks described in each scenario, the likelihood that these people with disabilities could complete such tasks was as follows (from the least likely to the most likely to complete the given tasks):

- Person on a wheelchair (S1)
- Person with a mild mental health condition (S2)
- Person suffering from alcoholism (S4)
- Person abusing substances (S5)
- Person with hearing impairments (S3)

These same people with disabilities were thought to encounter varying levels of difficulty doing these same ten tasks (ordered below from most difficulty to least difficulty):

- Person on a wheelchair (S1)
- Person with a mild mental health condition (S2)
- Person suffering from alcoholism (S5)
- Person abusing substances (S5)
- Person with hearing impairments (S3)

Concept mapping matrix and pile sorting

Items needing clarification

Items were translated into Arabic, but participants had difficulty understanding the exact definition of 36 of the 90 items. Examples of the difficult items include "Using special means of communication," "Keeping appropriate physical contact and maintenance of social space," and "Use of humour."

Items whose use in society is difficult for cultural reasons

Two concepts were thought be difficult to use for cultural reasons: sexual functions and performing consensual sexual acts.

Concepts not applicable for specific age groups

Several items were considered to be problematic for use in all age groups. These included economic self-sufficiency, managing a dangerous environment, expressing empathy, taking care of pets, cooking, sexual activities, using public transport, and responding to dangers.

Concepts understood differently by men and women

In total, 27 items were thought to be understood differently by men and women. Items in this category include dressing, leisure, work, planning/organizing meals, keeping rules/abiding by decisions, and taking care of the household.

Cultural sensitivity (taboo)

Five items were thought to be culturally sensitive: managing close personal relationships, managing relationships with friends, dating and forming relationships, sexual functions, and performing consensual sexual acts.

Focus groups

The two focus groups (health professionals and disabled people/families) provided similar input on the importance of the different domains of disability. Both groups saw the importance of the following domains: understanding and communicating with the world around you, getting around, self-care, getting along with people, and life activities. Conversely, both groups felt that the domain "Participation in society" was not of great importance and could be eliminated.

Conclusion

In Tunisia, parity does not exist among all causes of disability. Individuals with mental or substance-related disabilities are discriminated against more than those with disabilities due to physical impairments. Despite some problems with terminology and the applicability of concepts to all societal sectors, the overall ICIDH-2 conceptual model of disability is culturally appropriate and meaningful in Tunisia.

Chapter 17
Turkey

Aygün Ertugrul, Berna Ulug, Ahmet Gögüs, Kültegin Ögel,
*Defne Tamar, and Necati Dedeoglu**

Highlights from the CAR study in Turkey

- In Turkey, people with physical or cognitive disabilities are reported to encounter less stigma and discrimination against social participation than individuals with alcohol and drug problems.

- Drug or alcohol dependence are not considered as "diseases" in the community.

- In Turkey, disability is often judged and evaluated in the context of severity.

- The Government provides some services (special education, occupational rehabilitation, assistive devices, residential facilities, etc.) for physically and mentally handicapped people but they are not sufficient to meet the demand.

- Volunteer groups and associations have an important role in informing the Government of the needs of disabled people.

- Measurement of disability may be helpful in dealing equitably with the different disease groups and in determining the needs of disabled persons.

* Hacettepe University Medical School, Department of Psychiatry, Ankara (A. Ertugrul; B. Ulug; A. Gögüs); Bakirköy State Mental Hospital for Mental and Neurological Diseases, Istanbul (K. Ögel; D. Tamar); Akdeniz University Medical School, Dept. of Public Health, Antalya (Necati Dedeoglu), Turkey.

Introduction

Turkey is a southwestern Asian country with a population of 63 million. The CAR study was conducted at three sites: Ankara, Istanbul and Antalya. All these sites are big cities, with populations of 2.5, 10 and 1.5 million, respectively. The data reported are mainly based on urban populations so they may have some limitations in reflecting the views of the rural areas representing 40% of the country. Life expectancy is 68 years for male and life expectancy is 73 years for female; 36% of the population is under the age of 16.

In Turkey 60% of the population is covered by one of three government-owned social schemes:

- State Retirement Fund (for government employees);
- Social Insurance Agency (for insured workers);
- Fund for the Independently Employed (for artisans, professionals, etc.).

These schemes cover the insured together with their dependents. Workers who are not insured by their employers, farm workers and the unemployed have no social security.

Those covered are well supported by the system in the event of disability. Support includes medical treatment, institutional care, provision of devices, cash benefits and occupational rehabilitation. Wage and income compensation is available for temporary incapacity of employers or workers. If disability persists and is over 60% of working capacity, the person is given early retirement. It is illegal to dismiss a worker or employee on the basis of work incapacity for health reasons, mental disorders included. However, retirement pensions are insufficient and sheltered workplaces do not exist. Assessment and certification of disability are done in terms of capacity for work and are linked to the appraisal of eligibility for disability benefits and rehabilitation services. Percentage of capacity (e.g., a 30% loss of capacity for work) is used as a measure of disability, with ranges of percentages corresponding to the size of pension granted. An official commission consisted of five physicians from a local hospital is responsible for the certification of disability. A list prepared by Ministry of Health, which shows the percentage of loss of capacity for physical and mental disorders, is used for assessing physical and mental disabilities. If loss of capacity is greater than a certain proportion, a report is prepared stating that the person is unable to work and should be dependent on an insured family member or relative.

In both the workers' and state employees' insurance, if the disability is the result of a work accident or is considered by doctors to be an occupational disease, the disabled person is given preferential benefits and compensation. If not at the community level, at least legally there is parity between physical and mental disorders (excluding drug use and alcohol dependence).

Any privately or state-owned workplace with more than 50 workers is obliged by law to employ a specified proportion (3%) of disabled persons and exconvicts. The mentally disabled can also benefit from this law. Unfortunately, even Government establishments are unwilling to employ disabled persons when there are millions of healthy unemployed people and no supervision.

Methods

Instruments

The Turkish centre completed the following components of the CAR study: (1) key informant interviews, followed by the self-administered questionnaire; (2) pile sorting; and (3) concept mapping.

Sample

For the key informant and self-administered questionnaire studies 15 subjects were interviewed. They included three medical professionals, four allied health professionals, three policy-makers or opinion leaders, two people with physical health conditions or their care-givers, and three people with ADM (alcohol/drug/mental) health conditions or their care-givers.

The mean age of key informants was 40.2 (SD=10.9), with an age range of 22-58 years. Eight subjects were female and seven were male. The mean values for length of education were 13.7 years for females (SD=4.23)and 15.2 years for males (SD=5.22). Of the 15 people who were interviewed, six reported ever working in the field of physical disabilities, seven reported ever working in the field of mental disabilities, and six had ever worked in the alcohol/drug field.

Regarding the length of residence in the region, the respondents in Ankara, Istanbul and Antalya reported mean periods of 29.8, 20.4 and 8.2 years, respectively. For the concept mapping matrix and pile sorting study, a total of 30 subjects were recruited. Five respondents were medical professionals in the field of physical disability, 10 were medical professionals in the field of mental disability, five were people with physical disabilities or their care-givers, and 10 were people with mental disabilities or their care-givers. In total 22 females and 8 males were interviewed. The mean age of the sample was 40.23 (SD=9.6) with an age range of 24–57 years. Females had a mean of 16.1 years of education (SD=3.87) and males a mean of 16.3 years (SD=6.19). Eleven reported ever working in the field of physical disability, 13 in the field of mental disability, and eight in the field of alcohol and substance abuse. Seven subjects reported ever having a physical disability, six ever having a mental disability, and six ever having an alcohol/drug use-related problem.

The three sites shared three domains of disabilities. Ankara was the site for mental disabilities, Istanbul for alcohol and drug problems and Antalya for physical disabilities. Each site conducted interviews with 10 respondents consisting of five health workers and five consumers or care-givers. Subjects were recruited by focused and convenience sampling procedures. Consumers and care-givers were selected from a group of patients and family members at inpatient or outpatient units at the sites:

1. Department of Psychiatry, Hacettepe University School of Medicine, Ankara;

2. Clinics of the Centre for Alcohol and Drug Abuse Research and Treatment, Bakirköy State Mental Hospital, Istanbul;

3. General Hospital, Akdeniz University School of Medicine, Antalya.

Procedures

Key informant interview study

The interviewers in Ankara and Istanbul were psychiatrists. In Antalya the interviews were conducted by public health professionals. The interviews began with an introduction to the aims of the study. The responses were written down by the interviewer. The self-administered questionnaire and rank-order task were done immediately after the interview. Respondent information and the context of the interview were reported on the face sheet.

Concept mapping and pile sorting study

The instruments were briefly described to the subjects. The concept mapping matrix was given in a self-report format. Subjects reported their answers on a table. The glossary was presented to them in textual form. Thus cognitive debriefing could not be conducted for the negative responses. Subjects rated the first eight questions as either "yes" or "no." The last two questions were rated according to the printed scale. For the pile sorting study the same subjects sorted the cards without any intervention or help from the interviewer. Afterwards, the interviewer asked about the names the subjects had given of the piles and the reasons for the clusters they had created.

Results

Key informant interview and self-administered questionnaire

Quantitative analysis

Stigma ratings
Of the 17 health conditions presented, the three most stigmatizing conditions were drug addiction, alcohol problems, and criminal record for burglary. Drug addiction and alcohol problems are perceived more negatively than burglary. This indicates that, for people in general, disease concept of drug addiction and alcohol problems does not exist. The least stigmatizing conditions were being wheelchair-bound, being unable to read, and being blind.

Public reaction ratings
Being eight months pregnant, being obese and being blind are not met with disdain in public eye. Being visibly on drugs, being visibly drunk and being dirty and unkempt were the three conditions that attracted the harshest public reactions.

Rank-order of disability
The three conditions that were considered to be most disabling were quadriplegia, dementia and paraplegia. The three that were considered to be least disabling were infertility, vitiligo on the face, and severe migraine.

Activities
The key informants were asked to indicate how surprised people in their culture would be if persons with various conditions performed various activities. When the average scores were calculated across all 10 activities the order of conditions from being least likely to most likely to elicit surprise was as follows: person in wheelchair, person who hears voices, person with alcohol problems, person born with low intelligence, and person with heroin use problems.

When respondents were asked how likely it was that such persons would face barriers or restrictions in attempting to perform the activities, the order from least likely to most likely to face barriers was: person in a wheelchair, who hears voices, with alcohol problems, born with low intelligence, and with heroin problems.

Qualitative analysis

Qualitative analysis of the interviews revealed that in the Turkish culture the terms "disability," "handicap" and "impairment" are widely used interchangeably.

Key informants agreed that physical, mental and substance use problems all create difficulty in obtaining employment or getting married and having a family. They also emphasized that those with mental, alcohol and substance use problems have the most difficulty in doing a productive job and establishing positive relations in a family.

Regarding the difficulties of people with physical disabilities and mental retardation, some respondents blamed the poor social support system and inadequate accommodation of the public environment as the main cause.

Almost all respondents indicated that those with alcohol and drug problems do not deserve social assistance. For mental health problems, it was reported that degree of "severity" of the disorder is the factor determining the need for social assistance.

Disabilities from birth or caused by an accident were seen as deserving sympathy and mercy, and were considered as "fate" by some of the respondents. If alcohol or drug problems started after the death of a family member, the people concerned deserved more tolerance according to key informants.

Concept mapping and pile sorting

Problematic items and dimensions for Turkey

Needs clarification
* Interacting with an equal/co-worker/peer (item)
* Managing general psychological demands (item)
* Psychomotor activity (item)

Difficult to use in culture
* Thought, abstraction, judgement and related executive functions
* Using special means of communication
* Keeping appropriate physical contact and maintenance of social space
* Use of humour

- Activities related to fulfilling of financial obligations and services
- Dating and forming relationships
- Sexual functions
- Performing consensual sexual acts

Not useful for all age groups
Forty-nine items were reported as "not useful for all age groups." These results were not considered reliable.

Usability for all socioeconomic groups
- Using special means of communication
- Understanding specific signs
- Following written instructions
- Cultural activities
- Written communication
- Managing general psychological demands
- Activities related to fulfilling of financial obligations and services
- Dating and forming relationships
- Performing consensual sexual acts

Applicability for ethnic-minority groups
- Civic and community life
- Citizenship responsibilities

Cultural sensitivity of items
- Keeping appropriate physical contact and maintenance of social space
- Dating and forming relationships
- Sexual functions
- Performing consensual sexual acts

Classification of items into the levels of impairment, activity or participation
- Transferring oneself
- Community
- Seeing

- Mobility
- Civic and community life
- Hearing
- Citizenship responsibilities
- Moving around
- People sharing living space

Conclusion

In Turkey, people with physical or cognitive disabilities are reported to encounter less stigma and discrimination against social participation than persons with alcohol and drug problems.

The most stigmatizing health conditions were reported to be drug addiction, alcohol problems and a criminal record for burglary, whereas being wheelchair-bound, being unable to read and being blind were least stigmatizing. It is also interesting that in Turkey, though parental attitudes have great importance, someone who does not take care of his or her children is reported to attract less stigma than an alcohol- or drug-dependent person. Being visibly under the influence of drugs, being visibly drunk, and being dirty and unkempt were likely to be considered "wrong" in our culture. All the key informants indicated that people with alcohol and drug problems do not deserve social assistance.

These results show that drug and alcohol problems are not considered as "diseases" in the community. People with alcohol and drug problems are viewed as personally responsible for making these choices. Those with substance use problems seem to face more barriers to participation than people with other health conditions in Turkey.

The key informant interviews revealed that people consider mental health conditions and substance use problems more disabling and problematic. Obtaining employment, getting married and having a family were thought to be more difficult for these groups. Supporting the views reported by key informants, epidemiological research in community and clinical settings reveal strong correlation between mental disorder and impaired occupational and social functioning. In a WHO study, primary care patients with ICD-10 mental disorders reported greater occupational and physical disability than patients without a mental disorder (Ormel et al. 1994).

Spitzer and co-workers (1995) examined the association between broad mental disorder groups and impaired functioning. After controlling for other mental and general medical disorders, they found that anxiety and mood disorders were significantly associated with impaired social and role functioning. Sheehan, Harnett-Sheehan and Raj (1996) also showed that disability was high in psychiatric patients who often suffer more productivity impairment than patients with many chronic medical illnesses. Olfson et al. (1997) examined mental disorders and disability amongst patients in a primary care group practice and showed that individual mental disorders have distinct patterns of psychiatric co-morbidity and disability in Turkey. Some studies examining disability in the psychiatric population have also been carried out. Gögüs (1981) showed that chronic schizophrenic patients were significantly more disabled in all areas than acute schizophrenics, neurotics and a control group. In another study conducted in a primary health care clinic in a semi-rural area, patients with mental disorders were found to have more disability than patients with chronic physical disorders (Kaplan 1995).

In Turkey, disability is often judged and evaluated in the context of severity and assessed and certified in terms of capacity for work. The percentage of loss of capacity is used as a measure of disability, with ranges of percentages corresponding to the size of pension granted. An official commission composed of physicians is responsible for certification of disability. No strictly standardized instruments, procedures or criteria are used for disability. Determination of disability is often conceived only in terms of questions such as whether the patient can work or not. If not, should he or she be retrained, offered a sheltered job, or given a lifelong disability pension? Impaired functioning and incapacity are the measures of what can be compensated.

The importance of severity was also reflected in the key informant interviews. Respondents reported that social assistance depends on degree of severity of the health problem especially when mental health problems are involved. In summary, the real or perceived severity of disability determines public opinion and compensation.

Another important point is that long-term impairments such as quadriplegia, dementia and paraplegia seem to be publicly accepted as disabilities. In spite of that public opinion, wage and income compensation for temporary incapacity (e.g., during or following a psychotic episode) is available to employees and workers. A time limit exists for receiving benefits for what is termed temporary incapacitation (sick leave). There are differences in application between civil servants and workers under the social security system (up to three years for state employees, whether in hospital or on sick leave; for other workers some reduction of benefits after six months). If this period of sick leave has elapsed and the individual is not yet able to work normally or is in need of continuing financial support, an application for a disability pension is required.

We must also emphasize that although psychotic disorders and amnesic syndrome due to psychoactive substance use are considered to be disorders causing loss of capacity for work, alcohol and drug addiction or dependence is not included as a disability. This may be another result of the undeveloped "disease" concept for alcohol and substance use disorders. A review of the literature yields conflicting results on the degree of disability in alcohol and substance use disorders. Spitzer et al. (1995) showed that alcohol use disorders were not significantly associated with impaired role or functioning. In contrast, Olfson and co-workers (1997) found that substance use disorders were significantly associated with a composite measure of work, family and social disability. The relationship between alcohol dependence and disability has also been shown in the Turkish population (Berkasal 1981). Mercan and co-workers (1999) studied the impact of alcohol dependence on cognitive functions and social disability and showed that alcohol-dependent patients displayed significant neurocognitive impairment and high levels of social disability compared with healthy controls. It seems that more studies showing the relation between substance use and disability are necessary to form a strong basis before considering possible changes in the regulations on disability.

The key informant interviews, respondents reported that poor public accommodation makes the lives of disabled people more difficult. It is true that, compared with some developed Western countries, Turkey has few facilities for the disabled person. For example, there are few ramps for the wheelchair-bound and no braille signage for the blind. There are few schools for mentally retarded people.

The General Directorate of Social Services and the Ministries of Labour and Education provide some services (special education, occupational rehabilitation, assistive devices, residential facilities, etc.) for physically and mentally handicapped people but they are not sufficient to meet the demand.

Many volunteer groups, associations and foundations exist to provide community support to the disabled. Recently, the associations for the blind, deaf and other groups have organized themselves and formed a strong lobby. They have their own publications, TV programme and even disabled members in parliament. In 1986, associations for the blind, deaf, orthopaedically handicapped and mentally handicapped formed a confederation, named the Turkish Confederation of the Handicapped. This confederation organizes efforts to improve facilities and services for the disabled. It publishes a periodical in which it informs handicapped people about changes in regulations, employment facilities, and social activities such as sport competitions. The confederation also informs the government of the needs of the disabled people and problems in the application of regulations in real life.

Traditionally the disabled had always found support at the community level. Although rural areas still care for and make use of disabled people within the extended family, increasing urbanization and poverty have created new demands for institutional care and government support. In 1997, a Presidency for the Coordination of Disabled People's affairs was established in order to identify the problems of the disabled, find solutions for them, coordinate services for the disabled in a regular and effective way, and help to form a national policy on disabled citizens. In 1998, some changes were made to the tax law, reducing the amount of tax payable by disabled citizens and relatives who look after disabled persons. These are only some of the steps taken by the government to improve the lives of disabled people. No doubt there is much more to be done and studies on this issue will help to determine the new steps for the future.

In the concept mapping exercise, it was mostly items referring to activities and descriptions of participation relating to sexual function that were identified as culturally sensitive. This may be the result of the conservative structure of Turkish society. When interpreting the results of concept mapping, we also found that there was some difficulty in classifying items into the domaining of impairment, activity or participation, which shows that acceptance of these descriptions by our society will take time.

Chapter 18
United Kingdom

*R. Nichol and D. Mumford**

Highlights from the CAR study in the United Kingdom

- There is a felt need for greater public awareness and acceptance of mental and physical disability.
- Over the past 10 years, there has been a move to normalize facilities for people with disabilities.
- Successive governments over many years have been aware of the need to legislate to improve facilities for people with disabilities.
- Public anxiety about violence by people with mental health problems has increased, driven by stereotypes in the press and media.
- There has been a general move of people with different kinds of disability from residential institutions to community-based living arrangements.
- Mental health legislation is currently under review, particularly in relation to issues of consent to treatment.

Introduction

The data for this report were gathered from four cities in the United Kingdom (Bristol, Gloucester, Nottingham and Salisbury) in order to encompass a wide geographical area across England. The United Kingdom has a total population of 58.6 million people according to a 1995 estimate (England 48.9 million, Scotland 5.1 million, Wales 2.9 million, Northern Ireland 1.6 million). The percentage of the population aged under 16 years is 20.7%; aged between 16 and retirement age, 61.2%; over retirement age, 18.2%; and aged over 75 years 7.0%. Retirement age in the United Kingdom is at

* United Kingdom Centre, Division of Psychiatry, University of Bristol, Bristol, UK.

present 60 years for females and 65 for males. Table 1 provides a summary of the country's demographics.

Table 1. United Kingdom population figures, selected years, 1984–1995

Population group	1984	1993	1994	1995
Males (in millions)	27.5	28.5	28.6	28.7
Females (in millions)	29.0	29.7	29.8	29.9
Ethnic minorities	2,312,000	3,187,000	3,214,000	3,237,000

Source: Based on figures from the United Kingdom Government Office of National Statistics, 1998

Disability is recognized as a serious problem in the United Kingdom, and there are support services for a wide variety of disabling conditions. Table 2 provides demographic information on disabled persons living in residential facilities.

Table 2. Numbers of people with disability in residential care in the United Kingdom

Population group	1976–1977	1986–1987	1995–1996
Mentally ill in residential care (including elderly mentally ill from 1994–1995)	2,000	4,000	12,000
Elderly persons (over 65 years) in residential care	144,000	210,000	234,000
Young physically disabled people (under 65 years) in residential care	12,000	13,000	10,000
Residents with learning disability (mental retardation) in residential care	8,000	17,000	35,000

Source: Based on figures from the United Kingdom Government Office of National Statistics, 1998

The United Kingdom's financial support structure for disability is provided through three main sources:

- The State old age pension (available to those aged over 60/65 years);
- Unemployment benefit;
- The social security system, which provides basic income support plus a variety of specific financial benefits for disability.

There is also government legislation covering disabled persons, for example:

- *National Health Service Act, 1948*
- *Mental Health Act, 1983*

- *Social Services Act, 1970*
- *Disability Discrimination Act, 1995*
- *National Health Service and Community Care Act, 1990*

The present Labour Government is planning to refocus the social services system and revise the 1983 Mental Health Act during the next few years, in fulfilment of its election manifesto. This will have an impact on both definitions and services for persons with disabilities.

Methods

Instruments

The United Kingdom site completed all the basic components of the CAR study including the focus groups, but not the linguistic analysis. No additional concepts were included in the concept mapping exercise.

Sample

Pile sorting and concept mapping

Thirty subjects from a variety of backgrounds and from different geographical areas were interviewed. Of these, five were health professionals working primarily with physical disabilities; five were health professionals working primarily with mental health; 10 were consumers or care-givers primarily with physical disabilities; and 10 were consumers or care-givers primarily with mental disabilities. The sample was composed of 17 males and 13 females. The mean age was 41 years (males) and 42 years (females); subjects were drawn from a variety of health and other occupations. Table 3 provides additional information.

Table 3. Pile sorting and concept mapping: background of 30 subjects interviewed

Background	Currently	Previously	Never
Work or have worked with physical disability	9	6	15
Have or have had a physical disability	15	9	5
Work or have worked with mental disability	21	3	5
Have or have had a mental disability	1	7	22
Work or have worked with drug/alcohol	17	11	2
Have or have had a drug/alcohol problem	0	3	27

Key informant interviews

A sample of 15 people was selected at random for the key informant interviews, and to look at key concepts through the self-administered questionnaires. The sample consisted of three doctors, three nurses, two social workers, one health worker, three care-givers and three other professionals from a non-health occupation. There were six females (mean age 52 years) and nine males (mean age 42 years). Of the sample, seven were reported as working in physical disability, 12 in mental disability and 10 in drug and alcohol services, three had previously had experience with physical disability, and two had previous experience with drug/alcohol work.

Focus groups

In order to carry out the focus group study on parity and stigma of disabilities, two groups were selected. The first group consisted of health service users and some professionals drawn from the patients' council at a psychiatric hospital. The second group consisted of professionals and people with physical disability from a disability advice and drop-in centre. The first group included were members with drug and/or alcohol problems, although these people were not specifically identified. Within the second group, there were physically disabled people who had also suffered from mental health problems, although again they were not specifically identified. All members of both groups were volunteers and were guaranteed anonymity. The focus groups were tape-recorded and later transcribed, and some notes were taken during the group meetings. No formal consent form was used, but consent was obtained orally before each focus group meeting.

The focus group meetings were held at a psychiatric hospital and at a neighbourhood disability advice centre. Prior to the discussions, group members were informed of the subject area of questioning. The discussions were wide-ranging; however the interviewer endeavoured to focus the group on the questions to be addressed. As far as possible, direct quotations have been reported for each topic.

Procedures

No payment was made to any respondent, nor indeed requested, at any stage of the research. All interviews were conducted at participants' residence or place of work. Subjects were recruited through a networking process and asked individually if they would agree to participate in the research. All those approached appeared pleased to be asked and were given details of the study. Their agreement was sought twice, once on first contact, and again at the start of the interview.

One interviewer (RN) performed all the interviews for all parts of the study. It was felt that it was useful for one interviewer to carry out all the work because of the experience gained in procedures for administering the survey. On average the interviews lasted about two and a half hours.

Results

The words "impairment" and "retardation" are not used regularly in colloquial English. Mental retardation is usually referred to as "learning difficulties," and impairment can mean "handicap" or "disability/disabled." Information was provided in the focus groups about the lack of parity between mental and physical disabilities, in terms of stigma and services. One of the issues, summarized earlier, that emerged from a number of interviews and the focus groups was the increasing societal belief that the mentally ill are responsible for an inordinate amount of crime and violence in the United Kingdom, including violence in schools and on the streets.

Key informant interviews

Principal comments on the four scenarios

Physical difficulties
Mobility problems and visual signs of being disabled were described and used to illustrate the way in which others see a physically disabled person. It was suggested by half those interviewed that physically disabled people are often seen as having a mental disability. If the physical disability was caused by a road traffic accident it was felt that people have difficulty in dealing with sudden injury and do not know how to treat the newly disabled person; they are embarrassed and can be patronizing. People who are innocent victims of road accidents are likely to receive more sympathy; but there would be little sympathy if drugs or alcohol are involved and the accident is seen as their fault.

Mental health problems
Many respondents felt that attitudes would depended on whether the person was taking medication. Individuals who remained on medication were viewed more positively than individuals who stopped taking medications or refused

to take them. Self-care and lack of social acceptance were seen as some of the difficulties faced by persons with mental disabilities. Many felt that the question about being born with a mental disorder was not an acceptable question for the research, because it violated their view of the issue. The issues of marriage and work were not seen to be major difficulties, but again the question of taking medication was seen as a major factor. These social factors varied in relation to compliance with therapy.

Learning disability/difficulties
Again difficulties in self-care were seen as a major problem for individuals who had learning disabilities, together with self-neglect. It was felt that any work would be low-paid and repetitive. Marriage and close relationships were likely to be more problematic for these individuals than for persons with physical disabilities.

Drugs and alcohol
Drug- and alcohol-related problems were associated by a large number of respondents with violence and aggression. These disabilities are seen as highly stigmatized. Participants described individuals with a total obsession with alcohol to the exclusion of all else, leading to loss of family, home and work. It was felt that to get married was not a problem, but a high percentage of marriages fail because the drinker is secretive, isolated and covers up his or her obsession with alcohol.

State benefits
A system of State benefits is in operation in the United Kingdom. For people with learning disability (mental handicap), therefore, the question of benefit availability was not felt to be applicable in that country.

Degree of social disapproval

Of the 18 conditions presented, the four least stigmatizing were (in ascending order) being blind, being wheelchair-bound, depression, and borderline intelligence. The four most stigmatizing were (in descending order) drugs, criminal behaviour, not taking care of one's children, and alcohol.

Rank order of disability

The three most disabling conditions were considered to be quadriplegia, dementia, and (somewhat surprisingly) depression, which were ranked above being blind. The least disabling were infertility, vitiligo on the face and (surprisingly) HIV infection, with migraine coming next.

Social reaction

Of the conditions listed the most socially unacceptable was drunkenness, closely followed by being dirty and having a chronic mental health problem (acting out). The least social reaction was thought to be caused by pregnancy, being wheelchair-bound or being blind.

Pile sorting and concept mapping

Pile sorting

The pile sorting exercise was conducted, but during the process a universal problem in the use of language on the various cards was noted. Several respondents commented that the language on the cards and in the description was very American. The majority of participants appeared to have difficulty in seeing the relevance of the headings to the study. There were comments that the many of the concepts seemed too abstract, such as "recognizing," which several had difficulty placing. The researcher analysing the piles was able to recognize some of the respondents' beliefs, such as their attitude to religion and sexual matters, from the ways that they piled items together and labelled the piles.

Concept mapping

The concept mapping exercise. with the 10 questions, was criticized by all participants as being too long and time-consuming. After the initial interviews, it was found easier to devise an answer sheet and for respondent to read the various concepts and tell their answers to the researcher, who recorded them on a score sheet. Many of the questions were found to be too long; they could have been simplified into one general question which, depending on the answer, could have been used to probe for additional answers when necessary. It also became irrelevant to answer the rest of the list once participants had decided that a concept needed more clarification.

Focus groups

This part of the study uncovered some of the most interesting views from the participants and warrants further development in its own right. The results are summarized below under brief descriptive headings.

Attitudes and stigma

The groups felt that the public perception, often fuelled by the press, is that people with mental disorders are violent. In contrast, the participants considered that the mentally disabled were more likely to be the victims of violence from other members of society than perpetrators of violence. These are some quotations from the focus groups: "There is a lot of stigma for people with mental health problems getting jobs. Often there is evidence of them being turned down for jobs simply because they were honest enough to admit to having used the services." "Even the attitude of professionals is condescending to people with physical disability. We want to be treated normally but often if you are in a wheelchair you are seen as being simple-minded." "If you get the label of schizophrenia, that's the kiss of death really."

The following quotation from a member of the group with an alcohol problem sums up how many people in both groups felt: "I'm an alcoholic in recovery and that's going to be with me for the rest of my life. I accept it but other people don't accept it. I'm working to the best of my ability to control that but the outside world doesn't quite see it like that. We're back to stigma. I think in the type of job I would probably go for, I would have to hide this fact on my application. You are also a user of mental health services and have the stigma of being an alcoholic in recovery. That's it for life, and there are only trusted people you share that with."

Laws and social programmes for mental health, and drug/alcohol problems

The existing laws are designed to provide assistance for all groups of disability but in practice services are very patchy because of lack of fiscal resources and disagreements between the National Health Service and the Social Services Department (both government-funded). Various voluntary groups and nongovernmental organizations also provide help. Two examples are provided by the participants in this project. The mental health group was drawn from a voluntary self-help group for people with mental health, drug- and alcohol-related disability. The other was a voluntary advice centre for people with physical disabilities staffed in part by disabled people. These examples are typical of other groups around the country. Others agencies include social groups, advice groups, and employment, housing and rehabilitation groups.

As will be seen form the first question, it was felt that some mental health problems carry more stigma than others. Schizophrenia, epilepsy and manic depression are examples of this: stress and depression were felt to be more socially acceptable. Both drugs and alcohol were viewed with varying degrees of acceptance. Class A drugs (e.g., heroin, crack cocaine) were felt to be least acceptable by both groups. While alcohol in limited quantities is seen as socially acceptable, no mental disabilities are seen as positive.

The following quotations come from group members: "The image needs to be changed as even a lot of staff here still have attitudes from the 1950s. Some nurses are terrible and still don't respect you as an individual." "It's incredible that every time mental illness is mentioned in the media, particularly the tabloid press, it's associated with violence."

Services and laws for persons with mental disability compared with physical disability

This topic produced a number of interesting views from the two groups: "In court a person for example giving evidence... and if it's shown that this person has been a psychiatric patient, then their evidence is somehow diminished. Your rights are sacrificed as a result of a label being placed upon you." A mental health user felt that it might be easier to obtain work if a person has a physical disability. "If someone was in a wheelchair, people can see his or her problem and I would have thought it was easier for them." However, this was at variance with some other members of the mental health group and the physical disability group, who disagreed.

Another user thought there might be some advantages to physical rather than mental disability: "Employers might say, 'Well, it's just a physical disability. The job requires people to use their minds and their minds are obviously OK, so we'll give them the job'. With mental health problems they feel that their minds must be suspect, no matter how good their qualifications are, so they might write us off and give the job to a wheelchair user."

The physically disabled group, however, felt that it was harder because people can see the disability. "If people use the mental health services, they can hide that in their applications – we can't hide as we are sat there in a wheelchair. I personally think that people in wheelchairs face discrimination that is just as bad, if not worse, than mental health service users."

Changes necessary in society

The main theme was that society as whole needs to have further education and more understanding of what it is like to have a mental or physical disability. Both groups considered that there was a need to educate the public so that there is a much greater understanding of mental or physical disability.

Conclusion

The general theme was that while some services are available, they need to be expanded, facilities need to improve, and there needs to be a greater public awareness and acceptance of the difficulties faced by people who are physically and mentally disabled. This could possibly be done through school education to teach children more about the problems facing the disabled. The issue of parity for mental and physical disabilities will also have to be addressed in programme of this type.

Over the past 10 years there has been a move to normalize facilities for people with disabilities. It was suggested in discussion that this process has both benefits and negative consequences which should be explored in relation to evolving public policy. There has also been a move to place disabled persons in community-based rather than centralized residential institutions, in an attempt to provide services closer to families and homes.

The feeling was that at present there is a particular stigma attached to mental health disabilities. Too much of this is generated by the media, especially the tabloid newspapers, linking violence with mental health. It was considered that the situation for people with mental health problems would be relieved if there were a publicity campaign to show that mental illness can be successfully managed in the vast majority of cases.

Successive governments in the United Kingdom have been aware of the need to legislate for improvements in facilities for people with disabilities. Mental health legislation is currently under review, especially in the area of consent for treatment. However, both groups felt that service providers and professionals do not listen to the views of the disabled as a whole. Further work is needed on physical access to housing, workplaces, and public buildings for physically disabled people. The disabled themselves should make sure that the accessibility and facilities are suitable.

PART 3

CROSS-CULTURAL RESULTS

Chapter 19
Cross-Cultural Views on Stigma, Valuation, Parity, and Societal Values Towards Disability

R. Room, J. Rehm, R.T. Trotter, II, A. Paglia, and T.B.Üstün*

The CAR study was designed to provide empirical data on the concept of disability, the cross-cultural elements of disability terms, and cultural values concerning disabilities. The study also covered within-culture approaches to assistance, the relative stigma associated with different disabilities, and the extent to which there is parity in the ways that cultures approach disabilities associated with different kinds of health conditions – physical, mental, and alcohol or drug-related.

The CAR study protocol was partially or completely conducted at 16 participating centres. The centres collected both qualitative data and precoded information to provide extensive data on the cultural relativity of the disability construct and on the categories that form the backbone of the ICIDH-2 revised classification, and of the associated disability assessment instruments.

This chapter provides a summary and analysis of the key informant data, focus group data, and centre description information. The information gathered by the centres shows both strong commonalities and significant cross-cultural variation in societal responses to disabling conditions.

Methods

The overall CAR study focused on 12 basic data needs. Eight of those needs are discussed in this chapter, and the remaining four needs are presented in Chapter 20. The needs addressed here are:

---

* Centre for Social Research on Alcohol and Drugs, Sveåplan, Stockholm University, Stockholm, Sweden (Room); Centre for Addiction and Mental Health, Addition Research Foundation Division, Toronto, Ontario, Canada (Rehm, Paglia); Department of Anthropology, Northern Arizona University, Flagstaff, Arizona, USA (Trotter); WHO, Assessment, Classification and Epidemiology Group, Geneva, Switzerland (Üstün).

1. To create a general description of the place and meaning of disability and disability programmes in local cultures;

2. To summarize informants' descriptions of the current programmes, and need for programmes, that serve populations with disabilities;

3. To explore cultural contexts, practices, and values concerning disability;

4. To establish information on the thresholds that determine when, culturally, a person is considered disabled;

5. To compare the relative importance of different types of disabling conditions in different cultures;

6. To collect data on the parity or lack of parity between disabilities associated with mental health, alcohol and drug problems, and physical conditions;

7. To investigate information on stigma attached to various types of disabilities; and

8. To explore alternative conceptual models for the classification.

Table 1. Matching methods with relevant data needs

Research methods (*Types of data collected*)	Research issues for project	Data needs
Centre description information (*qualitative*)	Current practices and needs for disability services; policy information on disabilities; values and cultural responses to disabilities; legal status of disability assistance	General description of the meaning of disability; description of the current programmes; cultural contexts, practices and values concerning disability; parity or lack of parity; exploring alternative models; identifying linguistic equivalences for conceptual transfer
Key informant interviews (*qualitative, ranking*)	Cultural contexts, practices and values relating to disabilities; perceived relative severity of different disabling conditions; comparison between different disabling conditions	Cultural contexts, practices and values concerning disabilities; thresholds of disabilities; relative importance of different types of disabling conditions in different cultures; parity or lack of parity; stigma attached to various types of disabilities
Focus groups (*qualitative*)	Conceptual integrity of ICIDH-2 model, and suggestions for modifications; exploration of current practices and needs; parity between mental, physical and drug and alcohol use-related disabilities	

As was described in Chapter 2, each of these needs was carefully matched with one or more of the CAR methods. One of the goals of this matching was to assure that multiple methods were used to approach each data need, and that each need was covered by at least two, and preferably more, methods. This methods-matching approach turned out to be very valuable in the overall conduct and analysis of the project goals and data sets. Table 1 presents the matches between the methods and data collection needs reported in this Chapter. Pile sorting and concept mapping results are described in Chapter 20.

The CAR research was conducted at 20[1] sites in a total of 16 countries. Table 2 describes the number of informants represented in the data collected by all sites for these methods.

Table 2. Numbers of informants or data collection and reporting sessions

Method	Total N (all centres)
Centre	15
Key informant[2] interviews	230 informants at 18 centres
Focus groups	22 focus groups at 7 centres

Results reated to global issues

The global issues examined in the CAR study, such as stigma, thresholds and the general meaning of disability in the local culture, are the key qualitative conditions explored across the centres and the data sets. Many of these issues had a shared cross-cultural and cross-national core on which the differ-

---

[1] The centres which completed all six data collection tasks included three sites in India (Bangalore, Chennai and Delhi), Japan, The Netherlands, Nigeria, Romania, and Tunisia. Tunisia was responsible for data collection in Egypt, so there was no separate centre narrative for Egypt. The centres which collected all of the data except the focus group data included Canada, China, Greece, Luxembourg, Spain, Turkey (with sites in Ankara, Istanbul, and Antalya), and the United Kingdom. The United States site (Flagstaff) did not collect key informant interview data or concept mapping data. The Cambodian site was a later addition to the field group and provided a centre description, key informant interviews, focus groups data and the revised item evaluation data set. The sites that collected focus group data included Cambodia, India (three sites), Japan, The Netherlands, Nigeria, Romania, Tunisia, and the United States (Flagstaff).

[2] "Key informants" were defined as those who, by virtue of their position and knowledge, can capture and reveal relevant cultural phenomena, especially on disability. Within each site, 15 informants were to be selected, composed of three individuals representing the following five groups: health professionals (e.g., physicians, psychiatrists, psychologists, nurses), allied health professionals (e.g., social workers, case workers), policy makers or opinion leaders in the area of disability services, persons with a physical health condition (or their care-givers), and persons with a health condition in the area of alcohol, drugs or mental health (or their care-givers).

ent groups agreed. However, there were also strong differences in the emphasis, the valuation, and the local reaction to disabilities that emerged in the cross-cultural data sets.

Perceptions of current practices and programmes

Some of the most powerful data on the availability of programmes to assist disabled persons were collected during the focus group sessions held at each site. Participants discussed the programmes that were available, those that were not available and should be, and the reasons why they felt the coverage and the gaps existed. As noted in Chapter 3, there were three possible focus group topics and question models. For this issue, the data from the current practices and needs focus groups were found to parallel and augment the data from the parity and stigma focus groups in many ways. Part of the data from both data sets is compared and contrasted below to answer both sets of questions that were asked.

The amount of information focus group participants had about the law and the availability of services varied widely from individual to individual and group to group, depending on their exposure to the law and the assistance systems. Health professionals often had limited knowledge of the overall social programme systems in their society. Individuals with disabilities, and their caregivers, knew the most about programmes, services, laws, and conditions, especially those directly related to the disabilities that affected them. They tended to be more knowledgeable in those areas than many of the health professionals, with the exception of persons who worked for specific disabilities services. Health professionals have extensive knowledge of the disabilities that concern their area of specialization, but have limited knowledge (and occasionally no knowledge) of the laws, social service programmes, or advocacy and self-help groups associated with various other disabilities.

The participants indicated that many of the laws and programmes on disabilities focus on categorical conditions. There are programmes for the blind, deaf, and physically immobile, and other special categories, such as individuals who have served in the armed forces. But there is frequently no comprehensive or integrative system that embraces all disabling conditions. As a result, in order to qualify for various social assistance or income support programmes, the disabled individual is assessed in terms of diagnostic categories, i.e., not in terms of the activities that he or she can actually perform, but in terms of the categorical impairments he or she has. These assessments can be incomplete, irrelevant, or sometimes harmful. People with disabilities confront what they believe are a range of conflicting and non-interacting programmes each with different selection criteria and different types of help on offer. There is also a clear disparity in services provided depending on the stigma attached to different disabilities. Disabilities associated with mental health conditions and addictions are the most stigmatized and the least likely to receive adequate services or funding across all of the cultures reporting on the CAR study.

The cultural context of disability programmes

Five scenarios describing different health conditions were presented to key informants, as the primary method to determine the social and cultural contexts associated with disabilities and disability programmes. After some other questions, discussed below, informants were asked whether people in their culture believed that someone with a serious problem of that sort should get social assistance from the State. Comparing their responses when the serious problem was associated with a physical, mental, or drug or alcohol disorder revealed the implicit social context underlying these judgements (see Table 3).[3]

A majority of informants in each culture answered "Yes, assistance should be provided" for a serious mobility problem and for activity limitations linked to a serious intelligence problem and a serious mental disorder. However, they had considerably more reservations about providing assistance for the intelligence and mental disorder than for the mobility problem; in most societies, a minority gave the answer "It depends on the cause of the problem and its severity." In over half of the societies, a majority said "No" to the provision of assistance for a serious alcohol problem, and in about half of the societies the preponderant response was also "No" also for a serious heroin problem. Behind the "No" responses was likely to be the perception that the alcohol or heroin problem was self-induced.

In a related fashion, many of the "Yes" responses added that the provision of social assistance should be conditioned on the person being in treatment and motivated to change. In the context of alcohol and drug problems, social support tended to be viewed as an incentive for the affected person acknowledging a "need for assistance" defined in terms of treatment. The formulation in terms of having a "need for help" in the case of alcohol or drug problems often points towards compulsory rather than voluntary treatment.

Table 3 provides evidence that there is a clear downward gradient in support for state income and other forms of social assistance in most soci-

---

[3] The example given of a physical health problem is "Having difficulty walking or getting around unaided." In most people's minds, and not without reason, a mobility problem is caused by a physical health condition. It should be noted, however, that as a disability, a mobility problem could also be associated with a mental health or drug- and alcohol-health condition.

eties from disabilities associated with a physical condition and those linked to mental impairments and alcohol and drug problems. Support is high for social assistance for physical disabilities, and at best limited for social assistance for alcohol and drug problems. Once again, in the latter case the support for assistance was often conditioned on the person seeking treatment.

The key informant summaries indicate that popular attitudes are not supportive of parity in social assistance between physical, mental and alcohol and drug disorders. Even in societies where a majority of informants reported that there is support for social assistance across the board (China and Japan), there were substantial minority views concerning the alcohol and heroin disorders, as well as a suggestion that official views often run counter to actual practice in many different societies.

The data suggest that a number of presumptions lie behind societal views on social assistance. The most important of these involves the issue of where responsibility for the condition lies. Uncontrollable drinking and heroin use are widely seen as self-induced, and cross-culturally there is less sympathy for social assistance where the disabling condition is thought to be self-induced. On the other hand, when the etiology of a condition (whether physical, mental, or relating to substance use) is unequivocally assigned to causes outside the individual's control, there is generally more sympathy for the person with the condition, and more cultural support for the provision of assistance at a societal level. In many societies, conditions ascribed to fate, luck, or genetics are viewed sympathetically, although even here the sympathy does not apply if the person is seen as having contributed to the bad luck by his or her own actions.

There is also a clear exception to this general finding of greater sympathy for conditions with causes external to the individual. People in cultures that maintain a strong belief that bad outcomes reflect bad behaviour somewhere in the past, whether by the affected person or by the person's family, are far less sympathetic to people whose disabilities have been present from birth. Nigeria provides the clearest example of this: a majority of informants said that a mobility problem or a mental disorder present from birth is viewed as a divine sign that the parents did something bad. Key informants noted this theme also in India, and stigma for the family from a presumed genetic defect was implied in Greece, Japan and Turkey.

The degree of stigma or social disapproval attached to a condition seems to be strongly related to a reluctance to support state social assistance. It might be expected that individuals who confront the greatest barriers to participation in society would be thought to be in the greatest need of social assistance. But our informants report otherwise: there is a reverse correlation between orderings on the impact dimensions of various disabilities and the

Table 3. Support for social assistance for five conditions

Scenarios:
(a) Some people have difficulty walking or getting around unaided as the result of a health condition.
(b) Some people have difficulty with the activities of everyday life because they were born with low intelligence.
(c) Some people have difficulty with the activities of everyday life because they are bothered by strange thoughts, and sometimes they cannot control their actions.
(d) Some people have difficulty with the activities of everyday life because of their drinking of alcoholic beverages. They seem unable to control how much they drink.
(e) Some people have difficulty with the activities of everyday life because they take heroin. They are unable to control the amount of heroin they take or how often they take it.

Would people around here think they should get [state social assistance] if the problem was serious? – Yes; No; It depends.

Country	(a) can't walk	(b) low intelligence	(c) strange thoughts	(d) uncontrollable drinking	(e) uncontrollable heroin use
Canada	Yes	Yes (depends on severity and whether family/friends can support)	Yes (depends on degree or seriousness of problem)	It depends on severity and if in treatment (no, because it was own choice to drink)	Yes, but the person must be in treatment (no, because self-inflicted, depends on severity of problem)
China	Yes (depending on degree)	Yes (depends on severity)	Yes (sympathy, because of harm to self and society)	Yes (6 said no)	Yes (6 said no)
Greece	Yes	Yes (but some people do not care)	Yes, if a serious problem, (it depends, less popular support for mentally ill than for physically ill)	No (it depends, treatment but no financial help, 5 said yes)	Yes (no, it depends, treatment but no benefits)

Country					
India	Yes (depends on the individual & need, whether because of war or military service, depends on financial need)	Yes (depends on economic status, independent of economic status, no)	Yes (depending on seriousness, no, depending on financial status)	No (but treatment help, assistance to family, yes "people see this problem differently and are moralistically judgemental about it")	No (only treatment help, yes family members need assistance, "de-addiction" assistance should be given)
Japan	14 said yes should get assistance (2 said depends on the case)	Yes (1 said "it depends")	All said yes should get assistance	(7 said yes; 5 said no; 4 said depends on severity of case)	Yes (1 said no; 1 said it depends; 2 non-responses)
Luxembourg	11 said yes (3 said it depends if the person shows goodwill, 2 said it depends – not if due to alcohol/drugs)	12 said yes; (1 no; 3 it depends on degree of dependence/family support)	7 said yes (1 no; others: it depends on people's knowledge about these diseases, on degree of dependence, if person considered "crazy")	9 said no (2 yes; 4 it depends, including whether seen as disease)	8 no (3 yes; 4 it depends)
The Netherlands	Yes	Yes (1 said no)	Yes (no more difficult for mental than physical cases, partly because of inconvenience/nuisance for those around)	No (when it's related to life events, when the person seeks treatment, 2 said yes)	No (yes, yes with conditions)
Nigeria	8 said yes	7 said yes (no, it depends: more assistance in better educated/higher status communities)	Yes (8/15 no, it depends on whether seeking help/self-induced)	No (yes, it depends if looking for help, on severity of problem)	8 said yes (7 said no)
Romania	13 said yes (2: it depends on the degree of impairment)	Yes (1 said it depends on severity)	Yes (14/15 said it depends on severity & treatment access)	No (yes, it depends on somatic complications)	No (4 said yes)

Spain	Yes	Yes (2 said yes if unable to work)	Yes (if not able to work)	[both professionals and patients split on "yes" or "no because self-induced"]	[both professionals and patients split between "yes" and "no because self induced"]
Tunisia	Yes	Yes	Yes	No	Yes (majority; if stops/isolated, no)
Turkey	Yes	Yes (if serious)	Yes (majority; it depends on tolerance in family/on diagnosis)	No	No (majority; if motivated and severe, yes)
United Kingdom	13 said yes (it depends on whether wanted)	Yes, (1 said it depends on ability to work or receive family support)	Yes (9/15; 5 said it depends on response to treatment)	7 said no (6 said it depends on attitude to treatment, 2 said yes)	[missing data]

reported enthusiasm for state social assistance. There is strong support across the board for social assistance for a person with a mobility problem. In most societies social participation was more expected and less constrained for this condition than for any of the other four conditions.

The influence of etiology on judgements about disabilities

As a follow-up to the questions on social assistance, the key informants were asked whether the etiology of the problem would affect "how others thought of the problem and how the person was regarded." For the scenario on walking difficulty and "strange thoughts," respondents were then asked if it would make a difference to peoples' attitudes if the condition had been present from birth, and if it had resulted from a road accident. Table 4 summarizes the responses across centres.

In most societies it was felt that both of these etiologies would produce more understanding and sympathy than otherwise. However, in Nigeria it was felt that the presence of a problem from birth would further stigmatize the person, rather than lessen stigmatization; it would be felt that the affliction must be a curse from God. A minority of informants in Greece, India and Japan also mentioned that the affliction would cast aspersions on the parents or the person's genetic heritage (family prestige). And some informants in the United Kingdom felt that in this circumstance it would be assumed that there must also be a mental disorder associated with the other conditions. So, while the overall result was that these conditions were not strongly stigmatized, interpretations in some cultures could cause them to be stigmatized.

There were some other variations from the general tendency of responses concerning the impact of etiology on a mobility problem (first two columns of Table 4). A majority of informants in China felt that the fact that the mobility problem resulted from a road accident would not bring more sympathy. In India, a minority felt that the blame would actually be increased in this case with the occurrence of the accident being seen as a reflection of the person's past sins. In several societies (Canada, Japan, Luxembourg, The Netherlands, Romania, United Kingdom) a minority of the key informants mentioned that there would be more sympathy only if the circumstances of the accident made the person an innocent victim; in Canada and the United Kingdom, informants specifically mentioned that there would be no sympathy if the accident was seen as caused by the person's drinking or drug use. A few informants in Canada and the United Kingdom also mentioned that attitudes to the accident victim would be influenced by perceptions of who caused the accident.

Table 4. Influence of etiology on how problem was viewed: mobility problem v. mental disorder

What if the problem was something the person had had from birth – would that affect how others thought of the problem and how the person was regarded? In what ways?
What if the problem resulted from a road accident – would that affect how others thought of the problem and how the person was regarded? In what ways?

Scenario:	(a) can't walk		(c) strange thoughts	
Etiology:	If from birth	If from road accident	If from birth	If from road accident
Canada	Great pity and sympathy	Great pity and understanding if the accident was not the person's fault; but not if caused by person's drinking/drug use	Less blame, would not affect regard, would be lower expectations	Would not affect regard, pity and sympathy for their loss, depends on cause of accident
China	8 yes affected – more sympathy & help (7 no, would not affect)	11 no would not be affected (4 said yes, more sympathy)	10 said no effect (5 said yes, it would affect – more despised, more stigma)	8 said no effect (6 said yes, it would affect positively, in terms of compensation, public opinion, sympathy; 1 said yes, stigma)
Greece	Negative effect from stigma for family, would not affect attitudes, would increase sympathy	Negative effect since regarded as responsible for problem, increase sympathy, no effect	Would not affect regard, would bring more stigma, would bring more toleration	Would increase toleration; would make no difference
India	More sympathy and understanding (no difference, considered a burden/ sign of parents misdeed, sign of fate or supernatural punishment)	More sympathy and understanding (no difference, blamed more because of the accident, pity but also blame, fate, problem due to person's past sins)	Better understood and helped (will be rejected more, considered odd or an outcast, considered negatively as a curse or fate)	Sympathy and pity (more acceptance, less sympathy – considered worthless, will not change attitudes, considered as fate)

Japan	More sympathy (our society should help, genetic problem, bad luck)	More sympathy, no difference (bad luck, depends if victim or cause)	More sympathy, genetic problem, would not happen (avoid family)	Sympathy because it could happen to anyone, rarely happens (depends on the accident)
Luxembourg	More comprehension (no difference, risk of transmitting to children, more pity, feel helplessness, problem is more important)	Yes (depends if person's fault, no)	No difference (easily accepted, definitely classified, pity, person used to it, can happen to anybody)	Yes more easily accepted (pity, depends if person is responsible, no difference)
The Netherlands	Yes, positively; more compassion/understanding/acceptance (no)	Yes, positively (more compassion/pity where cause is outside the person, no, it depends)	Yes, more sympathy (no)	Yes, attribution to external cause brings more tolerance and compassion (no)
Nigeria	Worse if from birth – he is a sinner, the parents did something, it is a curse from God (more sympathy)	More sympathy – the family is not stigmatized because it could happen to anybody (it depends-could be seen as retribution for misdeeds, no difference)	Worse attitude (8/15 – "sent from the devil," act of God; greater sympathy, no influence)	More sympathy – could happen to anybody and "not as a result of someone's own faults."
Romania	10 more tolerance (3 worse, a real handicap)	9 more tolerance (4: the same; 2: it depends on the circumstances of the accident)	Worse attitude (9/15; more indulgent, no change in attitudes)	More indulgent – 7/15; no change in attitudes – 7/15; worse attitude
Spain	[Sample split on whether more compassion, less, or no difference if problem is from birth]	[Sample split on effect; detailed information missing]	More indulgent attitudes if from birth (no change)	[Missing data]
Tunisia	Acceptance (it's a matter of destiny), try to adapt (pity)	Feel solidarity, accept the situation (poor acceptance of the situation)	Getting used to the situation, it's one's destiny, support of family	Feeling of solidarity (mistrusting the person)

Turkey	No effect – 6/15; more sympathy – 5/15; less sympathy – 4/15	Some say will affect feelings, some not; most agree the situation is the person's fate	More sympathy and mercy (most; more anxious because will think hereditary)	More sympathy/fate/mercy/help (14/15; no effect)
United Kingdom	No effect – 4/15; protectionism/patronizing/sympathetic – 5/15; stigmatizing – 3/15; "If physically disabled, it is assumed must have mental disability" 7/15	More sympathetic if innocent victim – 7/15; no sympathy if caused accident through drugs or alcohol – 6/15; stigmatize – 3/15; no effect – 1/15	Split responses; 3/15 sympathetically, 5/15 less sympathy/exclusion/wary	More sympathy if innocent party – 7/15; less sympathy if from drink or drugs – 3/15

The key informant responses were very mixed in their interpretations of the influence of birth or an accident as the etiology of a serious mental disorder (Table 4, third and fourth columns). For a mental problem seen as being present from birth (which a couple of clinicians pointed out was unlikely for the mental problem as described), the balance of informants' views in Nigeria and Romania tipped toward thinking that it would produce a more negative attitude. Informants' responses on this were split in Canada, Greece, Luxembourg and the United Kingdom. In China, a majority said that this etiology would make no difference. Only in India, Japan, The Netherlands, Spain and Turkey did clear majorities say that more sympathy would be given to individuals who had this type of condition from birth, or after an accident.

On the other hand, where the problem resulted from a road accident, there was a clear majority that there would be more sympathy in Greece, India, Japan, The Netherlands, Nigeria, Tunisia and Turkey. In Canada, Luxembourg and the United Kingdom, opinions on this were split, as they were in relation to sympathy towards a problem that was present from birth. Again, the proviso that it depended whether the person was seen as responsible for the accident was mentioned in Canada, Japan, Luxembourg and the United Kingdom. Informants in The Netherlands and Nigeria specifically mentioned that being able to attribute a condition to an external cause brings more sympathy because the problem is then seen as one that could happen to anyone and is not "a result of someone's own fault."

This theme of personal responsibility became vividly apparent in responses to the scenario on an alcohol and a heroin problem. Informants were asked what difference it would make if the behaviour was seen as resulting from a death in the family (Table 5). We had hypothesized that such an etiology might be seen as potentially exculpatory for the condition in cultural situations where it was otherwise stigmatized.

The key informants' responses demonstrated that the stigma responses were sometimes modified or reduced in intensity from general disapproval, but there is a very clear message that compassionate or tolerant attitudes were conditional on whether the person voluntarily sought help or accepted involuntary help. The impression is also given that sympathy might not be long lasting. If a serious alcohol or heroin problem was seen as resulting from a death in the family it would generally produce more sympathy and tolerance, but not in Tunisia for either alcohol and heroin, nor in Canada, China, Luxembourg and The Netherlands for heroin.

The findings of this analysis underscore the fact that the terrain of disability, touching as it does on the whole gamut of daily life, is heavily influenced by social attitudes, including moral views. Beneath the varying degrees of

Table 5. Influence of etiology on how problem was thought of: alcohol and heroin problems

What if the problem was seen as being the result of a death in the family – would that affect how others thought of the problem and how the person was regarded? In what ways?

Country	(d) Uncontrollable drinking	(e) Uncontrollable heroin use
Canada	More sympathy and tolerance, but only for a certain period afterwards	No effect on how others thought, "no excuse" for using heroin (some sympathy, but only for short period)
China	8 said yes would affect – more sympathy (7 said no would not affect)	10 said no would not affect (5 said yes – more sympathy)
Greece	More positive attitude in this case, but only for a short period (would not really make a difference)	More positive attitude (but only for a while, makes no difference, less toleration than for alcohol)
India	More sympathetic, but only as a temporary problem (no change, just an excuse, it's a bad habit)	More sympathy, but only for the short term (no difference, not if it engages in antisocial acts)
Japan	[Missing data]	[Missing data]
Luxembourg	Tolerance and compassion for only a short time (no difference, more pity)	Makes no difference (3 said more tolerance, 2 said "yes," 1 said "depends on the drug")
The Netherlands	More understanding pity (but with a time limit, no effect)	No effect on other's view (should not react by taking drugs, yes on a temporary basis or because of external cause)
Nigeria	Greater sympathy (9/15; no sympathy)	Greater sympathy (9/15; no effect)
Romania	More compassion (13/15; no effect)	More compassion (12/15; no effect)
Spain	[Responses split]	["Better tolerated for alcohol than for drugs"]
Tunisia	A negative view no matter what the reason (pity)	Negative reaction whatever the reason (acceptance at first, then not)
Turkey	Greater mercy and tolerance (most)	More mercy and tolerance (majority)
United Kingdom	Yes (more sympathetic 4/15, yes for a short period; 5/15; no 2/15)	[Missing data]

stigmatization of different disabilities found in all the societies studied, there are undoubtedly culturally informed prejudices. There are also judgements about the moral status of the disabled person that reflect deeply felt views of how lives should be lived and how the social order should be constructed. Though a classification of disability must be etiologically neutral, in the sense of not presuming causal connections between health conditions, impairments, activity limitations and participation restrictions, it is clear that attitudes about etiology and presumed causal history determine many of the societal attitudes towards disability, and consequently towards any programme of assistance that will be developed to reduce the global impact of disability. These responses must be factored into the equations for understanding disabilities across and within cultural systems.

Cross-cultural variation in perceived thresholds of disabling conditions

Almost universally, the CAR centre reports indicated that having a systematic way of establishing the level, or threshold, at which disabling conditions should receive societal assistance was a common need. The reports also indicate that there is cultural variation about where these thresholds should be drawn.

An earlier cross-cultural applicability study of alcohol and drug disorders (Room, Janca, Bennett et al. 1996; Schmidt & Room 1999) demonstrated that there was considerable variation between cultures in the thresholds at which behaviours or conditions are noticed at all or are defined as problematic. These variations potentially affect cross-cultural epidemiological comparisons and have wider implications for health status and service utilization.

To make matters more complicated, thresholds can exist at various levels. There is the threshold of a condition being noticed. There is also the threshold where a condition is identified as a disability. In everyday social behaviour, occasional awkwardness, slowness or difficulty in behaviour or demeanour may not be noticed at all, or may not be called a disability. Whether and how stiffness in walking, breaking off and restarting sentences, or a minor facial tic is noticed is subject to variation both between and within cultures. Then, there may be additional substantial variation between cultures in terms of the levels at which a condition is viewed as a matter of some seriousness. Perceptions of seriousness may reflect aspects of the physical and social environment, as well as the level of individual impairment. What might otherwise be a serious problem may become much less serious when functional aids or environmental modifications are routinely available, or when eccentricity or other minor variations in personal style are readily accepted in a particular culture.

The key informant interviews explored the issue of thresholds by means of five anchor scenarios[4]. In each scenario, a health-related condition was said to cause difficulties with the activities of everyday life. The five scenarios were described as follows:

1. *Mobility problem:* "Some people have difficulty walking or getting around unaided as the result of a health condition. Sometimes their difficulty with this is obvious, but sometimes it is not."
2. *Mental disorder:* "Some people have difficulty with the activities of everyday life because they are bothered by strange thoughts, and sometimes they cannot control their actions. Sometimes their difficulty with this is obvious, but sometimes it is not."
3. *Low intelligence:* "Some people have difficulty with the activities of everyday life because they were born with low intelligence. Sometimes their difficulty with this is obvious, but sometimes it is not."
4. *Alcohol problem:* "Some people have difficulty with the activities of everyday life because of their drinking of alcoholic beverages. They seem unable to control how much they drink. Sometimes the difficulty with this is obvious, but sometimes it is not."
5. *Heroin problem:* "Some people have difficulty with the activities of everyday life because they take heroin. They seem unable to control the amount of heroin they take or how often they take it. Sometimes the difficulty with this is obvious, but sometimes it is not."

For each scenario, the respondents were asked three questions about thresholds:

a) If someone had a problem like this, but it was quite mild, what aspects of the person's behaviour might first attract the attention or notice of others, such as family members, neighbours or co-workers?
b) What if the problem was fairly serious – what would people consider to be signs of that (i.e., a serious problem)?

---

[4] The questions on thresholds were included in the key informant substudy of the CAR study. The present data analysis includes data from 11 countries. At the other sites, either insufficient data were collected, or they were summarized into English in insufficient detail for the present analysis. Each participating centre was asked to interview 15 key informants with an instrument combining questions with closed-ended codes and open-ended questions. For information about how key informants were selected see note 2. In India, three sites participated in the study. The actual number of key informants interviewed in each country is as follows: Canada 15, China 15, Greece 15, India 47, Luxembourg 16, The Netherlands 13, Nigeria 15, Romania 15, Tunisia (including Egypt) 15, Turkey 15, and the United Kingdom 15.

c) What would people consider to be signs that this person needed help from someone else with the activities of everyday life?

The wording of the first question was intended to introduce a minimum threshold, implicitly below the levels tapped by the other two questions. No assumption was built into the wording of the questions concerning the relative levels of severity of the second and third questions, although the fact that the question about needing "help from someone else" was placed third might have been assumed to imply greater severity. "Needing help" with a disability obviously implies an investment of human resources, whether paid or unpaid. In cultures placing a high value on individual autonomy, it may also be a dividing line infused with social meaning.

The responses to the questions about the mobility problem scenario most often started from the cue built into the question ("difficulty in walking or getting around"). There was fair agreement across the cultures that the threshold of attracting attention or notice includes such visible signs as slowness, stiffness, or limping. Unsteady balance was also mentioned at four sites (Canada, China, India, and The Netherlands). Informants in most countries focused on these physical signs, but some key informants mentioned that their culture also recognized psychological signs (nervousness and irritability – Greece, acting childishly – The Netherlands; avoidance of moving – Romania and United Kingdom; and looking for help – The Netherlands and Nigeria) that were associated with this threshold level.

The threshold between notice and seriousness was often demarcated by the use of an assistive device such as a stick, wheelchair, or other technical assistance. Differences in the availability of technical aids in some areas also produced mentions of "moving on all fours" or that the affected person "has to crawl." Falling or an injury were mentioned in five societies (Canada, India, Luxembourg, The Netherlands and Romania). While in China psychological sequelae (changes in consciousness, committing suicide) were mentioned in this context, in several societies (Canada, Greece, India, Nigeria, Romania, Tunisia, and United Kingdom) limitations in self-care activities were mentioned as criteria for establishing this threshold level.

The threshold for needing help was primarily answered by the respondents first assuming that help was needed and then listing the types of help that would be provided. This response made the identification of the threshold more difficult, and less clear. At five sites (Canada, Greece, The Netherlands, Romania, United Kingdom), respondents mentioned that the fact that a person asked for help was a sign that the person needed help. Answers from China and Nigeria implied a higher degree of disability for needing help than for a serious problem, mentioning paralysis or being unable to change positions. Most answers kept to a description of physical limitations that were associated with this threshold level. There were just a few mentions of psychological factors that could be associated with this threshold level (frustration, anger, or depression – United Kingdom; danger – Romania).

The mental disorder threshold for attracting attention or notice was defined by the presence of "out-of-context or inappropriate" social behaviours. These behaviours tended to relate to "irrational talk and behaviour," as a Nigerian respondent put it. Dangerousness (including aggression and hostile moods) was included by a number of informants from several countries: Greece, India, The Netherlands, Nigeria and Romania.

Several versions of "strange and odd behaviour" or talk were mentioned in most cultures as the salient criterion for identifying a serious problem. A notable criterion for establishing the threshold of a serious mental disorder almost everywhere (except The Netherlands) was aggression, violence, or harming others. In a majority of sites, poor self-care or being dirty or unkempt were also mentioned as criteria for identifying a serious problem.

The responses for the threshold of needing help were similar to, but more extensive than, those associated with the threshold of identifying a serious problem. The threat of aggression or harm to oneself was a prominent theme in a majority of cultures. Neglect of self-care was also mentioned in a majority of cultures, although informants in China and Tunisia focused more on impaired communication and comprehension. Asking for help was mentioned in fewer societies (India, The Netherlands, and the United Kingdom) than for the mobility problem. Overall, the thresholds for serious problems and individuals needing help were virtually identical for mental problems.

The low intelligence threshold scenario produced many responses that focused on childhood slowness or retardation. The threshold for noticing this condition was the most clearly dependent on age, and the comments about intervention tended to be age-specific as well. Difficulties in communication were mentioned as one sign of impairment by informants from many cultures, but the pattern of responses suggests that the threshold for this condition may be set at a more extreme level (only noticed when a person cannot communicate at all) in China than elsewhere. The focus of the threshold recognition conditions was on cognitive disabilities, but there were also some mentions of difficulties in social functioning (China – no sense of shame; India – silly behaviour; Romania – childish behaviour; Nigeria – unkempt, abnormal behaviour) as part of the recognition process.

Little differentiation is made between the threshold of notice and the signals of a serious problem for low intelligence in many cultures. The cognitive dimensions of functioning figured in most answers concerning a serious problem, but an added element of the responses from many sites was a dimension of dangerousness or social deviance added to the other conditions. Aggression or temper tantrums were mentioned in the responses from Canada, India and The Netherlands; other responses pointing in this direction were added by other sites: lacking a sense of danger (China); causing accidents or fires (Turkey); coarse or inappropriate demeanour (Tunisia); and indulging in vices (Nigeria).

At nearly all sites, the criteria for identifying the threshold of where when help is needed included problems in self-care or in performing basic activities. But in conjunction with this, a majority of informants in all societies mention a dimension of dangerousness to others or lack of a sense of danger to oneself (China, Greece, India, Romania), of aggression or anger (India, Tunisia, United Kingdom), or of a lack of judgement or moral reasoning (Nigeria, United Kingdom) as key threshold criteria.

For the alcohol problem scenario, informants offered a variety of signs that might first attract attention or notice to an alcohol problem. Many of these are related to specific drinking-related behaviours or signs (e.g., slurred speech, smell of alcohol). These threshold conditions often carried the implication that it is the repetition of the behaviour that counts, not just a single instance or instances that were very far apart ("a lot of drinking" – China; "excessive drinking habit" – India). A dimension of compulsiveness or pre-occupation with use was mentioned in several sites (Canada, China, Greece, and United Kingdom). In a majority of sites the threshold of notice included poor performance in work or family role responsibilities. The idea of erratic behaviour or a change in behaviour was mentioned at several sites.

This was the first scenario that produced a clear pattern in which socially derogatory signs were identified even at the level of first notice of the problem. These included aggressiveness (Greece, India, Nigeria, United Kingdom), irritability (Romania), lying (India, United Kingdom), and vagabondage (Tunisia).

Responses from Tunisia emphasized physical and psychological signs to indicate a serious alcohol problem, along with "refusing advice" and "loss of conscience." At all other sites, neglect of major social roles was the key response, along with aggression and violence. Only four societies (Canada, Greece, India, and United Kingdom) included responses from key informants that identified physical health problems as signs that the problem is serious.

The criteria for needing help did not seem to differ greatly from the criteria for a serious problem in this scenario. A person's failure in his or her social roles and acts of violence was prominent in the identification of the seriousness of the problem, along with a variety of physical, psychological and social signs. Tunisian informants emphasized "danger to others" as a criterion, and this theme also appears more diffusely elsewhere (e.g., in Greece and India where there was mention of the family needing help). This response alerts us that "needing help" in some cultural contexts is socially defined in ways other than volunteering assistance to the person with disability. It can imply a societal demand for compulsory treatment for the individual as well as assistance to others who are affected by the person with the problem. In contrast to the first two scenarios, no site mentioned "requesting help" as a sign of needing help with a serious alcohol problem.

The primary emphasis in responses to the heroin problem scenario, on what would first attract attention or notice, was on behavioural and mood changes. Though some physiological signs were offered (e.g., "glassy eyes" – India; "scratching one's nose" – Tunisia), the main signs mentioned for a heroin problem were more generalized than for alcohol. Fewer sites mentioned aggressiveness or irritability, but lying (China, India) or secretive behaviour (Canada, Nigeria) were mentioned.

For the threshold signs for a serious level of impact, aggression was less commonly mentioned for heroin than for alcohol, although it was mentioned in Greece, India, Luxembourg, Nigeria and Romania. Involvement in criminal activities was often mentioned. Defaults in major social roles were somewhat less prominently mentioned than for alcohol. It is possible that there is less direct knowledge of the physical signs of heroin addiction among this set of informants, and therefore they had to rely on general social knowledge to be able to discuss the threshold scenario.

The criteria for needing help were, as with alcohol, not clearly distinguished from signs of a serious problem. At a majority of sites, lack of self-care or being dirty or untidy were mentioned; other recurrent themes were neglect of daily tasks and antisocial behaviours. "Danger for others" was explicitly mentioned only in Tunisia. As with the alcohol scenario, there was no mention of "requesting help" as a sign of needing help.

When the responses to all of the scenarios are compared, it is interesting that the key informants often did not give information that created very clear differentiation between the three thresholds of attention, serious problem, and needing help. This was especially true for distinctions between the thresholds for "serious problem" and "needing help": the answers to the two were either identical or only minimally distinguishable. With the exception of the scenario on mobility, dangerousness to self or others was often an element used to differentiate the threshold of notice and that of a serious problem. In responses to the need for help threshold, the added element was often failure in self-management of mundane activities. For the mobility scenario, and less commonly also for the mental disorder scenario, asking for help was mentioned as a sign of needing help.

Responses to both the alcohol problem and the heroin problem scenario usually emphasized morally defined signs, even at the minimum threshold of being noticed. The individual's failure to perform social roles, and aggression or violence, were commonly cited as signs of alcohol problems; with heroin, the emphasis was less on violence and more on secretiveness. For those with alcohol and drug problems, there is the added burden of the tendency to see the problem as voluntarily assumed; as one respondent from the Netherlands put it concerning indications for needing help for the heroin problem scenario, "no help because no sympathy." In contrast, while a person with a mental disorder or low intelligence may also fail to fill major social roles, this failure is not described as part of the problem, but as a consequence of the problem. At the far end of this spectrum, responses concerning restriction of mobility were not oriented to inherently negative social evaluations.

The responses of the CAR key informants suggest that the five problems asked about are widely defined in terms of a moral gradient, in which a physical mobility problem is the least negatively evaluated in social terms, and alcohol and drug problems are most negatively socially evaluated. The key informant responses for the mental disorder and low intelligence scenarios were generally less negatively socially assessed than responses for alcohol and drug problems. Only the physical mobility problem responses rarely contained a moralized dimension in all cultures. The intensity or steepness of the moral gradient varied across cultures. The differential across the five scenarios seems somewhat less in Canada, for instance, than in India, but the existence and direction of the gradient is clearly evident in responses from every society.

The relative importance of disabling conditions: The ranking exercise

A substudy within the CAR key informant study addressed the question of how different cultures rank or rate the seriousness of different disabling conditions (this study is reported in Üstün, Rehm, Chatterji et al. 1999). From the perspective of the CAR research, it was important to discover whether there were any meaningful differences in the ranking of the disabling effects of health conditions by key informant from different countries. It was also of interest to discover whether different informant groups (medical professionals, allied health professionals, health policy-makers, consumers or caregivers) rank health conditions in meaningfully different ways.

Key informants from the participating countries were presented with a deck of 17 cards listing different health conditions (see Chapter 3 for details). They were asked to rank the conditions from the most to the least disabling. The "most disabling condition" was described as that which would make daily activities very difficult; the "least disabling" was described as that which would not interfere with the activities of everyday life. Numerical codes were assigned to the 17 conditions, with "01" representing the most disabling, and "17" representing the least disabling.

Non-parametric statistics for ordinal-level variables were used to analyse the data. Overall ranking was established on the basis of the median. Health conditions with the same median were ranked using the arithmetical mean as the second criterion. To test for differences between countries or informant groups, Kruskal-Wallis rank order analysis of variance for one factor was used. Spearman and Kendall Tau B correlation coefficients were computed to measure the association between different rank orders.

Table 6 gives an overview of the relative rank order for the 17 health conditions, ranked from most disabling to least disabling. Overall, quadriplegia was considered the most disabling condition across all cultures, followed by dementia (rank 2), active psychosis (rank 3), and paraplegia (rank 4). At the opposite end of the spectrum, having vitiligo on the face (least disabling = rank 17), being infertile when a child is desired (rank 16), and having severe migraines (rank 15) were deemed the least disabling. The conditions at both ends of the spectrum, that is the most disabling and the least disabling conditions, showed lower variability than the conditions in between (see standard deviations in Table 6).

There were deviations from this combined measure of order within countries. Table 7 shows that in The Netherlands and Canada, for instance, active psychosis is seen as more disabling compared to the overall-sample rank, whereas in Tunisia it is seen as far less disabling. Being HIV-positive is considered relatively less disabling in Japan, Luxembourg, Spain, Turkey and the United Kingdom, whereas it is considered the most disabling in Egypt and Tunisia. HIV-positivity is, in general, the health condition with the most variation in rank (see also Table 6).

Statistically, the differences between countries were significant for 13 out of 17 health conditions on the Kruskal-Wallis test. Only quadriplegia, paraplegia, below-the-knee amputation and mild mental retardation did not show rank differences between countries at the 0.05 significance level. It is interesting to note that three out of the four conditions that are judged uniformly across countries are prototypical physical disabilities. The fourth, mild mental retardation, does not show the same degree of uniformity as the other three.

Although there are statistically significant differences of ranking between countries, the convergence of judgements is also quite evident. The Kendall Tau rank-order correlations between different countries averaged 0.615 and the Spearman rank correlations averaged 0.777, which can be considered relatively high given the variation among the cultures and experts participating. Within this average, there are clear cultural differences for some comparisons; for example Japan and Tunisia have a Kendall rank order correlation of 0.441 (Spearman: 0.581), or The Netherlands and Tunisia correlate at 0.294 (Spearman: 0.431). This would suggest that there are clusters of cultural viewpoints about disability rankings, and some cross-cultural agreement, but there is no universal vision of the ranks across all disabilities.

The rank-order ratings of different informant groups are summarized in Table 8. Only four out of 17 health conditions had significantly different rank orders between different informant groups: HIV positivity, total deafness, mild mental retardation, amputation below the knee. Interestingly, again physical disorders are the most prominent, but in this case as conditions with the most significant differences. HIV infection is the most variable condition in this study. It was ranked from the most disabling of all health conditions in Egypt and Tunisia to the third least disabling condition in Luxembourg. The differences among expert groups are less dramatic but still important. The differential availability of expensive treatment may contribute to these quite different judgements. In general, it can also be said that the physical condi-

Table 6. Rank order of disabling effect of health conditions by severity

Health condition	Rank	Median	Mean	Standard deviation	N
Quadriplegia	1	2	3.349	3.184	241
Dementia	2	4	4.896	3.648	241
Active psychosis	3	4	5.290	3.626	241
Paraplegia	4	5	5.938	3.262	241
Blindness	5	6	6.780	4.037	241
Major depression	6	6	7.224	3.821	241
Drug dependence	7	8	7.847	3.874	222
HIV positive	8	9	8.791	5.155	239
Alcoholism	9	9	9.237	3.553	241
Total deafness	10	10	9.411	3.705	241
Mild mental retardation	11	10	9.851	3.555	241
Incontinence	12	10	10.159	4.087	239
Below the knee amputation	13	11	10.249	3.736	241
Rheumatoid arthritis	14	12	11.531	3.629	241
Severe migraines	15	12	11.629	3.789	240
Infertility	16	16	14.630	3.569	238
Vitiligo on face	17	16	15.000	2.410	238

Table 7. Disability ranks associated to different health conditions by country

Health condition (in rank order of total sample)	Canada	China	Egypt	Greece	India	Japan	Luxembourg	The Netherlands	Nigeria	Romania	Spain	Tunisia	Turkey	United Kingdom
Quadriplegia (1)*	2	1	2	1	1	2	1	3	1	1	1	2	1	2
Dementia (2)	3	8	3	3	2	1	2	2	6	2	2	3	2	1
Active psychosis (3)	1	5	4	2	5	3	3	1	3	3	4	6	4	4
Paraplegia (4)*	4	4	8	4	4	5	7	7	2	4	5	4	3	5
Total blindness (5)	8	3	5	9	3	4	4	9	5	5	6	5	5	8
Major depression (6)	5	6	7	7	6	8	6	4	4	7	3	7	11	3
Drug dependence (7)	7	2	6	6	11	7	5	6	10	11	11	11	7	M
HIV positive (8)	10	9	1	5	7	13	15	12	8	8	8	1	14	14
Alcoholism (9)	9	10	11	8	10	10	8	5	13	13	13	12	10	6
Total deafness (10)	11	12	10	13	9	6	9	11	15	9	9	13	12	12
Mild mental retardation (11)*	6	11	9	12	12	15	10	13	11	10	10	9	8	7
Incontinence (12)	15	13	13	10	8	14	13	15	7	6	12	10	6	11
Below-the-knee amputation (13)*	12	7	12	11	14	9	11	14	12	12	11	8	9	13
Rheumatoid arthritis (14)	14	14	17	15	13	11	14	10	14	15	15	16	13	10
Severe migraines (15)	13	15	16	14	15	12	12	8	9	14	14	17	15	9
Infertility (16)	16	17	14	16	17	16	17	16	16	16	17	15	17	16
Vitiligo on face (17)	17	16	15	17	16	17	16	17	17	17	16	14	16	15
N	15	15	16	15	43	18	16	13	15	15	18	15	15	12

Note: Ranking ranges from 1 (most disabling) to 17 (least disabling). "Most disabling condition" defined as that which would make carrying out the activities of daily life very difficult; and the "least disabling condition" defined as that which would not interfere with activities of everyday life. M=missing data; item not given.
* No significant differences between countries on (P = 0.05 level).

Table 8. Disability ranks of different health conditions by informant group

Health condition (in rank order of total sample)	Medical professionals					Allied health professionals (N=51)	Health policy makers (N=35)	Consumers/care-givers	
	Physical (N=14)	ADM (N=35)	Physical and ADM (N=14)	Other (N=11)	Total (N=74)			Physical (N=36)	Mental (N=45)
Quadriplegia	1	1	3	1	1	1	1	1	1
Dementia	2	2	1	2	2	3	2	4	2
Active psychosis	5	3	2	4	3	2	3	2	3
Paraplegia	3	4	4	3	4	5	4	6	4
Blindness	6	5	5	5	5	6	7	5	5
Major depression	4	6	6	6	6	4	5	8	6
Drug dependence	9	7	7	8	7	7	9	7	8
HIV positivity	10	11	15	11	11	12	6	3	7
Alcoholism	13	10	10	9	9	8	10	9	9
Total deafness	12	8	9	7	8	10	11	11	12
Mild mental retardation	14	13	8	12	13	9	8	10	13
Incontinence	7	12	14	13	12	11	12	12	11
Below-the-knee amputation	8	9	12	10	10	13	13	13	10
Rheumatoid arthritis	11	14	11	15	14	14	14	15	14
Severe migraines	15	15	13	14	15	15	15	14	15
Infertility	16	16	17	16	16	16	17	17	16
Vitiligo on face	17	17	16	17	17	17	16	16	17

tions are ranked more uniformly and universally than mental conditions across countries, but not across informant groups.

Parity or lack of parity among health conditions

WHO has an international mandate to seek to create parity among health conditions. Parity is the goal of ensuring that society's health and related resources are provided to people according to their health requirements, not solely in terms of whether the underlying health condition can be characterized as a "physical" rather than a "mental" or "alcohol or drug abuse" health problem. In many of the countries involved in the CAR study, parity has not yet been achieved. Health insurance policies differentiate between whether the acquired condition is physical, mental or related to substance abuse; social benefits are allocated differently according to etiology and category of health condition. Even anti-discrimination provisions, in those countries that have them, often only apply to people whose disability is not the result of an alcohol or drug disorder.

The data from the CAR focus groups clearly indicate that in all the cultures sampled there is a stark lack of parity (both in the assistance provided and in attitudes towards individuals with disabilities) between physical, mental and alcohol- and drug-related disorders. Groups of health professionals, persons with disabilities and their families all unanimously agreed that a wide variety of negative social attitudes are common towards individuals labelled as mentally ill, or those with alcohol or drug problems. These are not as commonly directed towards persons with purely physical health conditions. Those who readily expressed their culture's compassion, understanding and willingness to accommodate people with physical health conditions often went on to note the culture's impatience, disdain, or even outright hostility towards alcoholics and mentally ill people. The most often cited basis for this difference was the extent to which the health condition is a result of voluntary actions or morally culpable behaviours. In the case of mental illnesses, most participants in the focus groups reported the cultural view that such individuals are unpredictable and probably dangerous.

A question on parity posed to the focus groups was whether, in their view, the services and laws applicable to persons with mental health problems are equal to those applicable to persons with physical health problems. Many participants were able to cite examples in their society where services and legal protections available to people with physical conditions were not available or less readily available to those with mental health conditions. A member of the focus group in Nigeria noted that much of the country's legislation does not clearly apply to mental illness; and a participant in a Bangalore focus group pointed out that the Indian policy of job reservation quotas for persons with disabilities does not apply to those with mental health problems. In the United Kingdom focus group several participants thought that their country's rights protection legislation did not adequately cover the rights of people with mental health problems.

Significantly, when participants said that they were unaware of the social services available to people with disabilities, or the precise coverage of laws designed to protect their rights, they still did not hesitate to say that the policies and laws of their culture make a distinction between physical and mental health conditions. They cited differences in restrictions on the right to vote, run for office, or own property. The clear difference in social attitudes, they believed, made it self-evident that there would also be a difference in social policy and law.

Social disapproval or stigma

The data indicate that the majority of individuals in public and in the workplace avoid individuals with disabilities, and find it difficult to work with them. This discomfort increases significantly with mental conditions, and is very high with alcohol- and drug-related health problems. There is some individual variability, but for the most part persons with disabilities face high levels of workplace discrimination and avoidance. It was noted in focus groups that the families of individuals with disabilities often face the same stigma and avoidance. The disabled individual's prospects of marriage are greatly diminished and in those societies where marriage has retained many of its traditional function, other children in the family may also be denied the opportunity of an advantageous marriage.

In the CAR study, key informants were asked questions about a collection of health conditions and disabilities that would elicit data about their perception of the degree of social disapproval that individuals with these conditions would be likely to encounter in their culture. For comparison other, socially visible conditions or states were added: not being able to hold down a job, being dirty and unkempt, not taking care of one's children, having a criminal record for burglary, and being pregnant. Then questions were asked to elicit cultural information about expectations of what activities people with various disabilities should engage in and the likelihood that they would face social barriers to participation. The aim throughout was to operationalize stigma in ways that are relevant to disability.

Ranking of social disapproval

Key informants were first asked to report their understanding of the degree of social disapproval or stigma that people with various health conditions would encounter in their culture. Eighteen Likert-type rating scales were used to assess the level of negative reaction experienced by someone with each condition. The scales ranged from 0 (no social disapproval) to 10 (extreme). The 18 conditions are listed in Table 9.

Mean ratings of social disapproval were calculated for each condition. Since there was variation between sites in the actual ranges informants used in their assessments, the results are presented in terms of a relative ordering for each society. Across societies, those in wheelchairs, those who were blind, and those who could not read received the least amount of social disapproval, while those with alcoholism, a criminal record, HIV infection, or drug addiction received the highest level of disapproval.

Substantial differences in ordering were found in social disapproval ratings for obesity. In relative terms, obesity drew more stigma in Canada, Turkey, and the United Kingdom, and less in China, Greece, India, and Japan. Depression drew relatively high stigma in Japan and Tunisia, but relatively low stigma in China, Romania, Spain, and the United Kingdom. Being unable to hold down a job drew relatively less stigma in Japan, while homelessness was especially stigmatized in Canada, The Netherlands, and Romania. Leprosy drew a relatively high stigma in Nigeria and China, but low stigma in Tunisia. In Nigeria, leprosy was more stigmatizing than in Egypt and Tunisia. The social disapproval level for someone who does not take care of his or her children was relatively low in Turkey and Japan, but high in Egypt, Luxembourg, and Tunisia.

When each country's ranks are compared with the overall rank order, it can be seen that in Canada, obesity, homelessness and not taking care of children faced more disapproval, while alcoholism was met with relatively less social disapproval. In China, obesity, depression and not taking care of one's children are conditions that were less stigmatizing, whereas leprosy was relatively more stigmatizing. In Egypt, depression was regarded as relatively more, and homelessness relatively less, stigmatizing. In Greece, those in wheelchairs face more disapproval, and the obese face less disapproval. Japan's stigma ordering shows that those in wheelchairs, who are blind, or who have depression or a chronic mental disorder face more disapproval. On the other hand, those who are obese, have a facial disfigurement, are dirty and unkempt, or do not care for their children may trigger relatively less negative reaction in Japan. In Nigeria, those with a chronic mental disorder or leprosy seem to face more social disapproval. In Tunisia, depression was considered

Table 9. Degree of social disapproval or stigma relative ordering from lowest to highest mean rating within each country

Condition (in rank order of total sample)	Canada	China	Egypt	Greece	India	Japan	Luxem-bourg	The Nether-lands	Nigeria	Romania	Spain	Tunisia	Turkey	United King-dom
Wheelchair bound (1)	2	3	1	5	2	5	2	2	1	3	2	1	1	2
Blind (2)	1	5	2	2	4	9	1	1	3	1	1	2	3	1
Inability to read (3)	6	6	3	3	1	2	5	3	2	5	4	5	2	6
Borderline intelligence (4)	3	4	4	7	5	7	3	4	5	7	5	7	6	4
Obese (5)	9	1	5	1	3	1	4	7	4	4	6	3	14	11
Depression (6)	5	2	10	4	6	15	6	6	9	2	3	12	5	3
Dementia (7)	4	8	7	6	9	10	9	8	7	8	7	4	9	5
Facial disfigurement (8)	7	7	8	8	8	3	7	10	6	6	8	9	8	7
Cannot hold down a job (9)	10	11	12	10	10	4	8	9	11	10	11	11	7	10
Homeless (10)	16	9	6	9	7	12	13	15	8	16	10	8	12	8
Chronic mental disorder (11)	12	13	11	12	14	17	10	8	15	9	9	10	10	12
Leprosy (12)	11	16	9	15	13	11	11	11	18	13	14	6	13	9
Dirty and unkempt (13)	15	14	13	11	12	8	12	12	12	12	13	13	11	14
Does not take care of own children (14)	18	10	16	14	11	6	16	14	10	11	15	17	4	17
Alcoholism (15)	8	12	15	13	15	14	15	16	13	14	12	14	17	15
Criminal record for burglary (16)	13	17	17	16	16	13	17	17	17	18	16	15	15	16
HIV positivity (17)	14	18	14	18	17	16	14	13	14	15	18	16	16	13
Drug addiction (18)	17	15	18	17	18	18	18	18	16	17	17	18	18	18
N	15	15	16	15	47	18	16	13	15	15	18	15	15	12

Note: Ranking of 1 indicates least stigma, ranking of 18 indicates most stigma.

more stigmatizing than many other conditions, including dementia; leprosy was less stigmatizing than the average. In Turkey, the item "not taking care of one's children" did not provoke as much disapproval, whereas obesity drew relatively more. In the United Kingdom, obesity elicited more social disapproval than many other conditions, while being HIV-positive elicited relatively less social disapproval. India, Luxembourg, Romania, and Spain seemed to have mean orderings on stigma similar to the overall sample.

The sample of informants as a whole clearly indicated that physical disabilities – e.g., being confined to a wheelchair or being blind – carry the least social disapproval. The Japanese data deviated most substantially from this, but even here the conditions remain in the top half of the ordering. Infectious diseases that are potentially deadly or disfiguring – HIV and leprosy – drew considerably more disapproval, and are generally in the bottom half of the ordering, though leprosy elicited less disapproval in Turkey and the UK. A plurality of mental impairments or disorders – borderline intelligence, depression, and dementia – drew only moderate stigma, being generally in or near the top half of the ordering (depression is more stigmatized in Japan). Chronic mental disorder is at or below the middle of the list in most countries, and particularly stigmatized in Japan, Nigeria, and India.

Alcoholism and drug addiction were mostly strongly stigmatized (near the bottom of the list except for alcoholism in Canada) ranking with or below highly stigmatized social characteristics such as homelessness, being dirty or unkempt, or a criminal record for burglary.

The mean orderings on stigma in Table 9 in cultures with a close kinship – e.g., the UK, and Canada, and Luxembourg, and The Netherlands – were often similar. But otherwise it is difficult to discern clear clusterings of response. For instance, there is no clear differentiation in orderings between developing and developed societies.

Reactions to appearing in public

Informants were asked about public reaction to people with certain conditions appearing in public (e.g., on a bus, or in a store or market). The 10 conditions asked about are listed in Table 10. The six response options were:

1. People would think there was no issue, and would pay no attention
2. People would notice, but would not think there was any issue
3. People would be uneasy about it, but would probably not do anything
4. People would be uneasy about it, and try to avoid the person
5. People would think it was wrong and might say something about it
6. People would think it was wrong and try to stop it

Table 10. Public reaction: ordering from lowest to highest mean rating within each country

Condition (in rank order of total sample)	Canada	China	Egypt	Greece	India	Japan	Luxem-bourg	The Nether-lands	Nigeria	Romania	Spain	Tunisia	Turkey	United King-dom
A woman in her 8th month of pregnancy (1)	1	1	5	1	1	2	1	1	1	1	1	4	4	1
Someone who is blind (2)	3	4	4	2	4	3	3	3	4	6	3	2	2	2
A person in a wheelchair (3)	2	5	3	5	5	4	2	2	2	3	2	3	5	3
An obese person (4)	5	2	2	3	2	6	4	4	3	1	5	1	9	4
A person who is intellectually "slow" (5)	4	3	1	4	3	9	5	5	5	4	4	5	7	5
Someone with a face disfigured from burns (6)	6	6	6	6	6	1	6	6	6	5	6	7	3	6
Someone with a chronic mental disorder who "acts out" (7)	7	8	7	8	8	8	7	9	7	8	8	6	1	7
Someone who is dirty and unkempt (8)	8	7	8	7	7	5	8	7	8	7	7	8	6	8
Someone who is visibly drunk (9)	9	9	9	9	9	7	9	8	9	9	9	9	8	9
Someone who is visibly under the influence of drugs (10)	10	10	10	10	10	M	10	10	10	10	10	10	M	M
N	15	15	16	15	47	18	16	13	15	15	18	15	15	12

Note: The question was "Please indicate how people in this society would react to a person with the health condition appearing in public." A public reaction score is based on ratings from 1 ("People would think there was no issue, and would pay no attention") to 6 ("People would think it was wrong, and would try to stop it"). M=missing data; item not included in questionnaire.

In the analysis below, these six responses are treated as an interval scale, with a higher score indicating a greater disapproval of a public appearance.

Again, generally speaking, it is apparent that being in a wheelchair and being blind, along with being eight months pregnant, are not met with disdain in the public eye. Also consistent with the previous section is the finding that being dirty and unkempt, and being either visibly drunk or on drugs in public were likely to be considered "wrong" in some respect across cultures.

There is some variation in the rank orderings. In Egypt, for instance, a woman appearing in public in her eighth month of pregnancy received more criticism than, say, a person who is intellectually "slow." Similarly, in Tunisia being pregnant and appearing in public was slightly more "taboo." In Japan, someone who is "intellectually slow" would be relatively less accepted when appearing in public than elsewhere, while someone who is disfigured from burns would be more accepted. In Romania, someone who is blind would receive relatively harsher reactions for appearing in public. In Turkey, again, an obese person would be less accepted when appearing in public, while someone with a mental disorder who "acts out" would be relatively more accepted than elsewhere.

Table 11 presents a closer look at the extreme end of the distribution, showing the proportion of informants who felt that "people would think it was wrong" for the person with each condition to appear in public. As the relative rankings in Table 10 suggest, there is considerable variation in Table 11 between cultures in the proportion reporting that people "would think it wrong" for an obese person to appear in public. Other conditions showing substantial disagreement between cultures include someone whose face is disfigured from burns, someone who is intellectually "slow," and someone with a chronic mental disorder who "acts out." Japan, Canada, Turkey, and The Netherlands appear more tolerant than other cultures of someone who is visibly drunk or someone who is dirty and unkempt appearing in public. Only for someone who is visibly under the influence of drugs did a majority of informants in the sample say that "people would think it was wrong" to appear in public; Canada and The Netherlands also reported more tolerance than elsewhere for someone with this condition.

Level of surprise at and presence of social barriers

Key informants were presented with five scenarios designed to explore the presence of social barriers, based on whether or not people would be surprised that individuals with different conditions were engaged in specific activities. The scenarios included:

1. A person who confined to a wheelchair because of a spinal cord injury
2. A person born with low intelligence
3. A person who says there are voices talking to him or her all the time
4. A person who is in a bar constantly with a drink in hand
5. A person who is constantly under the influence of heroin

In order to gauge cultural expectations of what activities people with such health conditions can perform, informants were asked, for each of 10 activities: "How surprised would people be if this person did this activity?" Response options were "Not at all surprised," "A little surprised," "Surprised," and "Very surprised." Informants were also asked: "Is it likely that anyone would place restrictions or barriers on the person doing this?" Response options were "Very unlikely," "Somewhat unlikely," "Somewhat likely," and "Very likely."

Table 12 presents the overall percentages, aggregated across all sites, of the respondents who would be surprised (or very surprised) if they saw or heard about someone with a health condition doing the activities listed, as well as the likelihood that barriers would be encountered. There are substantial variations between different activities. Taking public transportation and having sex are activities which would be particularly surprising for someone in a wheelchair, but not for someone with any of the other conditions. A person born with low intelligence is believed to be likely to face barriers with regard to performing most of the 10 activities. The majority of respondents indicated that they would be surprised if someone who hears voices kept a full-time job or became elected to a government position.

A majority of respondents across countries indicated that someone with an alcohol or heroin problem would be unlikely to keep things tidy, take on parenting roles, keep a full-time job, or hold a position in local government. In addition, according to most respondents, persons with such problems would be likely to face some type of barrier in taking part in community festivals, becoming a parent, managing money, keeping a job, or becoming elected.

In Table 13 the ordering of the five conditions for "surprise" and "likely to face barriers" for each site is presented. These orderings are based on average scores calculated across all 10 activities for each country. For the sample as a whole, a person in a wheelchair ranked lowest on both "surprise" and "barriers faced," whereas a person who hears voices ranked highest. Canada is most notably different with respect to a person with an alcohol problem (which ranks in Canada as provoking the least surprise and facing the least barriers), and somewhat different for the low intelligence health condition. In China, persons with alcohol or heroin problems fared the worst. In Greece, people with mental

Table 11. Public reaction: percentage responding "People would think it was wrong" for a person to appear in public, by country

Condition	Total %	Country													
		Canada	China	Egypt	Greece	India	Japan	Luxem-bourg	The Nether-lands	Nigeria	Romania	Spain	Tunisia	Turkey	United King-dom
A woman in her 8th month of pregnancy	2	0	0	0	0	4	0	0	0	7	0	0	0	7	0
Someone who is blind	3	7	0	0	0	6	0	0	0	7	13	0	0	0	0
A person in a wheelchair	2	0	0	0	13	7	0	0	0	0	0	0	0	0	0
An obese person	12	20	7	13	7	6	19	31	8	13	0	17	0	20	8
A person who is intellectually "slow"	7	7	0	0	0	4	23	0	0	13	0	0	14	33	8
Someone with a face disfigured from burns	6	0	33	6	0	0	0	12	0	20	0	0	13	7	0
Someone with a chronic mental disorder who "acts out"	15	0	33	0	20	17	12	19	17	13	27	22	0	0	17
Someone who is dirty and unkempt	25	20	27	69	20	17	0	44	8	47	40	17	43	0	33
Someone who is visibly drunk	46	13	27	88	27	46	6	81	8	80	73	50	79	14	50

Someone who is visibly under the influence of drugs	58	20	57	100	40	67	M	56	17	64	67	56	79	M	M
N	245	15	15	16	15	47	18	16	13	15	15	18	15	15	12

Note: The question was "Please indicate how people in this society would react to a person with the health condition appearing in public." "Think it was wrong" refers to responses: "People would think it was wrong, and might say something about it" and "People would think it was wrong and try to stop it."
M=missing data; item not included in questionnaire.

Table 12. Surprise that a person with a health condition performs an activity, and likelihood that a person would face barriers (N=245)

Country	Person in wheelchair	Person born with low intelligence	Health condition		
			Person who hears voices	Person with alcohol problem	Person with heroin problem
Keeping things tidy					
Would be surprised	48	19	46	66	67
Likely to face barriers	43	15	32	24	26
Using public transportation					
Would be surprised	55	13	23	15	17
Likely to face barriers	49	28	45	37	39
Being in love					
Would be surprised	25	25	44	21	22
Likely to face barriers	45	53	62	46	50
Having sex (as part of a relationship with someone)					
Would be surprised	50	26	34	12	14
Likely to face barriers	45	56	59	38	42
Actively taking on parenting roles					
Would be surprised	28	48	60	49	64
Likely to face barriers	32	55	69	54	68
Actively taking part in community fairs and festivals					
Would be surprised	23	21	40	37	42
Likely to face barriers	26	32	58	55	60
Managing own money					
Would be surprised	6	68	40	37	42
Likely to face barriers	20	74	54	56	62

Getting an apartment or somewhere to live					
Would be surprised	18	46	42	24	36
Likely to face barriers	33	58	56	37	51
Keeping a full-time job					
Would be surprised	31	40	65	62	79
Likely to face barriers	39	49	72	65	73
Being elected or named to a position in local government					
Would be surprised	44	86	86	76	90
Likely to face barriers	49	86	88	82	90

Note: The questions and included responses were "How surprised would people be if this person did this activity?" – "Surprised " and "Very surprised"; and "Is it likely that anyone would place restrictions or barriers on the person doing this?" – "Somewhat likely" and "Very likely."

health problems (low intelligence, hears voices) seem to face the most obstacles. A person in a wheelchair in India and Nigeria was perceived as least likely to carry out the given activities, relative to the other conditions. In Egypt, Japan, Nigeria, Spain and Turkey, a person with a heroin problem seemed to be most likely to face barriers. In The Netherlands and Romania, this can be said for a person with low intelligence.

As already noted, issues of social disapproval and barriers to social participation were approached in the key informant interviews from several angles. In Table 14, the patterning of responses on these questions concerning each of five health conditions are summarized in terms of the relative ranking of the five conditions. This reflects the comparative emphasis of this analysis, and also steers around the apparent differences in the tacit systems of measurement used by informants at different sites.

Averaging across all sites, the person in a wheelchair – the physical health problems used as an index condition – was viewed as the least stigmatized and the most socially accepted to appear in public of the five conditions. In terms of social and daily-life activities, participation by the person in a wheelchair would also overall be the least surprising, and would meet the fewest restrictions or barriers. Second in terms of less stigmatization and more acceptance of appearing in public was the person with low intelligence, followed in order by the person with a chronic mental disorder, the person with an alcohol problem, and the person with a heroin problem. The ordering on participation in social and daily-life activities was somewhat different, with the person with an alcohol problem ranking second, the person with low intelligence third, and the person with a chronic mental disorder last.

In terms of the relative stigma of the five conditions, a majority of societies – Greece, India, Luxembourg, The Netherlands, Romania, Spain, Tunisia, Turkey, and the United Kingdom – followed the ranking of the average across sites. The other societies – Canada, China, Japan, and Nigeria – showed a minor deviation in ordering, the person with an alcohol problem less stigmatized than the person with a chronic mental disorder. In general, the convergence in the ordering of stigma among the conditions was impressive.

A number of societies – Canada, Luxembourg, Nigeria, Romania, Spain, Tunisia, and the United Kingdom – followed the same rank order as the average ranking across all sites for acceptance of the person with the condition appearing in public. For answers to this question, deviations in ordering were more varied. In China, Greece, and India, more acceptance was reported for a person with low intelligence appearing in public than for a person in a wheelchair. In Japan and The Netherlands, a person with an alcohol problem ranked higher than elsewhere on appearing in public. A person with

Table 13. Ordering of five health conditions by "People would be surprised" and "They would be likely to face barriers"

Country		Person in wheelchair	Person born with low intelligence	Health condition		
				Person who hears voices	Person with alcohol problem	Person with heroin problem
Total Sample	(order on) Surprised	1	3	5	2	4
	(order on) Likely to face barriers	1	3	5	2	4
Canada	(order on) Surprised	2	4	5	1	3
	(order on) Likely to face barriers	3	4	5	1	2
China	(order on) Surprised	2	1	3	4	5
	(order on) Likely to face barriers	1	2	3	5	4
Egypt	(order on) Surprised	1	3	5	2	4
	(order on) Likely to face barriers	1	2	4	3	5
Greece	(order on) Surprised	1	5	4	2	3
	(order on) Likely to face barriers	1	4	5	2	3
India	(order on) Surprised	4	1	5	2	3
	(order on) Likely to face barriers	1	2	5	3	4
Japan	(order on) Surprised	1	4	3	2	5
	(order on) Likely to face barriers	1	3	4	2	5
Luxembourg	(order on) Surprised	1	3	5	2	4
	(order on) Likely to face barriers	1	3	5	2	4
The Netherlands	(order on) Surprised	3	5	4	1	2
	(order on) Likely to face barriers	1	5	3	2	4
Nigeria	(order on) Surprised	3	1	4	2	5
	(order on) Likely to face barriers	2	1	4	3	5
Romania	(order on) Surprised	1	5	2	3	4
	(order on) Likely to face barriers	1	4	2	5	3

Spain	(order on) Surprised	1	2	4	3	5
	(order on) Likely to face barriers	1	2	4	3	5
Tunisia	(order on) Surprised	1	2	5	3	4
	(order on) Likely to face barriers	1	2	5	3	4
Turkey	(order on) Surprised	1	4	2	3	5
	(order on) Likely to face barriers	1	4	2	3	5
UK	(order on) Surprised	1	2	5	3	4
	(order on) Likely to face barriers	1	4	5	2	3

Note: The questions asked were "How surprised would people be if this person did this activity?" and "Is it likely that anyone would place restrictions or barriers on the person doing this?" Ordering is based on means. 1 = least surprised, and least likely to face barriers.

Table 14. Social disapproval, expectation of social participation, barriers to social participation: ordering of 5 health conditions

Country	Person in wheelchair	Person born with low intelligence	Health condition Person who hears voices	Person with alcohol problem	Person with heroin problem
Total sample (N=204)					
Degree of stigma (1=less)	1	2	3	4	5
Public appearance (1=OK)	1	2	3	4	5
Participation expected (1=more)	1	3	5	2	4
Participation barred (1=less)	1	3	5	2	4
Canada (N=15)					
Degree of stigma (1=less)	1	2	4	3	5
Public appearance (1=OK)	1	2	3	4	5
Participation expected (1=more)	2	4	5	1	3
Participation barred (1=less)	3	4	5	1	2
China (N=15)					
Degree of stigma (1=less)	1	2	4	3	5
Public appearance (1=OK)	2	1	3	4	5
Participation expected (1=more)	2	1	3	4	5
Participation barred (1=less)	1	2	3	4	5
Greece (N=15)					
Degree of stigma (1=less)	1	2	3	4	5
Public appearance (1=OK)	2	1	3	4	5
Participation expected (1=more)	1	5	4	2	3
Participation barred (1=less)	1	4	5	2	3
India (N=47)					
Degree of stigma (1=less)	1	2	3	4	5
Public appearance (1=OK)	2	1	3	4	5
Participation expected (1=more)	4	1	5	2	3
Participation barred (1=less)	1	2	5	3	4
Japan (N=18)					
Degree of stigma (1=less)	1	2	4	3	5

Public appearance (1=OK)	1	4	3	2	—
Participation expected (1=more)	1	4	3	2	5
Participation barred (1=less)	1	3	4	2	5
Luxembourg (N=16)					
Degree of stigma (1=less)	1	2	3	4	5
Public appearance (1=OK)	1	2	3	4	5
Participation expected (1=more)	1	3	5	2	4
Participation barred (1=less)	1	3	5	2	4
Romania (N=15)					
Degree of stigma (1=less)	1	2	3	4	5
Public appearance (1=OK)	1	2	3	4	5
Participation expected (1=more)	1	5	2	3	4
Participation barred (1=less)	1	4	2	5	3
Spain (N=18)					
Degree of stigma (1=less)	1	2	3	4	5
Public appearance (1=OK)	1	2	3	4	5
Participation expected (1=more)	1	2	4	3	5
Participation barred (1=less)	1	2	4	3	5
Tunisia (N=15)					
Degree of stigma (1=less)	1	2	3	4	5
Public appearance (1=OK)	1	2	3	4	5
Participation expected (1=more)	1	2	5	3	4
Participation barred (1=less)	1	2	5	3	4
Turkey (N=15)					
Degree of stigma (1=less)	1	2	3	4	5
Public appearance (1=OK)	2	3	1	4	5
Participation expected (1=more)	1	4	2	3	5
Participation barred (1=less)	1	4	2	3	5
United Kingdom (N=15)					
Degree of stigma (1=less)	1	2	3	4	—
Public appearance (1=OK)	1	2	3	4	—
Participation expected (1=more)	1	2	5	3	4
Participation barred (1=less)	1	4	5	2	3

low intelligence ranked lower than elsewhere on this dimension in Japan and Turkey. In Turkey, indeed, public appearance was reported to be most accepted for the person with a chronic mental disorder.

The responses from Canada were unique in ranking the person with an alcohol problem lowest both on surprise at, and on restrictions and barriers to, social participation. Other societies where the person with alcohol problems ranked relatively low on these dimensions included The Netherlands and Greece. On the other hand, it was reported that in China and Romania the person with alcohol problems would find the most restrictions on social participation, even greater than for the person with a heroin problem.

Altogether, in seven societies the person with a heroin problem was ranked lowest or next to lowest on social participation expectations and resistance, while this person would be met with relatively less surprise and resistance, it was felt, in Canada and The Netherlands. In most societies, social participation by the person in a wheelchair would be greeted with the least surprise and resistance. The surprise would be relatively greater in India and Nigeria; only in Canada and Nigeria were the restrictions or barriers on participation expected to be less for another condition than for the person in a wheelchair.

Overall, the ordering of the five conditions showed considerable variations across dimensions and across sites. Nevertheless, some general patterns emerge. Both on stigma and on expectations of participation, the person in a wheelchair is generally regarded the most favourably. For stigma, the persons with alcohol and heroin problems usually rank high, while for expectations and restrictions on participation, it is the person with a chronic mental disorder and the person with a heroin problem who generally vie for the least favourable position.

Summary and conclusions

The centre report, focus group, and key informant data made a significant contribution to the CAR study's ability to explore both cross-cultural comparability of views on disability, and the significant differences in the ways that individual societies attached stigma, evaluated the need for assistance, noticed the problem in the first place, and attached evaluations of severity to different kinds of health conditions. The results strongly indicated that the model of disability found in ICIDH-2 is sufficiently cross-culturally applicable to justify the continued development and dissemination of the international classification, and they solidly supported the current and future work on creating an international "language of disability."

The following chapter explores the structure of the classification of disabilities, and the specific concepts behind the conceptualization of disability that have been implicit in this chapter.

Chapter 20
The Structure and Stability of the Proposed International Classification

J. Rehm, R.T. Trotter, II, S. Chatterji, and T.B. Üstün*

Introduction

The data presented in this chapter had a direct impact on the content and structure of the ICIDH-2 classification, and the development of assessment instruments. The methods were chosen to help to identify the correct placement of items in the classification, and to present clear information on the cross-cultural stability of the structure of ICIDH-2 as a whole.

Methodologically, the data are at the other end of the spectrum from the data produced to investigate the more global issues concerning disability reported in the previous chapter (key informant, focus group and centre description data). While the data have significant qualitative components, the methods used are designed to provide a qualitative-quantitative bridge in the continuum of cross-cultural applicability methods. The primary question the methods were asked to answer was whether the concepts and items in the draft classification and assessment instruments could be constructed to include only items that met both the cultural and the psychometric requirements for the development of the classification and associated disability instruments.

Methods

The CAR methods chosen for this task were procedures that focused on individual elements of the classification, and the relationships of those elements to one another. The data needs identified for this section included:

* Centre for Addiction and Mental Health, Addiction Research Foundation Division, Toronto, Ontario, Canada (Rehm); Department of Anthropology, Northern Arizona University, Flagstaff, Arizona, USA (Trotter); WHO, Assessment, Classification and Epidemiology Group, Geneva, Switzerland (Chatterji, Üstün).

1. The need to identify linguistic equivalences for conceptual transfer of elements of the classification into local languages, and back into English;
2. To determine whether the proposed structure of the classification has good cross-cultural stability;
3. To provide an item-by-item evaluation of the cross-cultural applicability of each facet of the classification;
4. To collect data on the boundaries between the three domains of the classification system.

In addition, the methods were employed to gather further information on the potential cultural sensitivity of the items, and to compare the relative importance of different types of disabling conditions in different cultures. Table 1 presents the matches between the methods and data collection needs reported in this Chapter. It should be noted as well that the method selected not over covered these needs but also allowed a significant degree of triangulation of results, without unnecessary duplication.

Table 1. Matching methods with relevant data needs

Research methods (*Types of data collected*)	Research issues for project	Data needs by method
Translation/back-translation and linguistic analysis protocols (*qualitative*)	Linguistic equivalences for items or sections off the classification; identification of problematic individual items.	Identifying linguistic equivalences for conceptual transfer.
Pilesorting (*qualitative and quantitative*)	Cross-cultural stability of the classification; identification of problematic individual items; discovery of underlying cultural dimensions within the classification.	Investigating proposed structure of the classification; and item-by-item evaluation of cross-cultural applicability.
Concept mapping (*quantitative, some qualitative*)	Cultural applicability of items; problems with taboo; age and gender bias; socio-economic conditions; linguistic problems with items.	Cultural contexts, practices and values concerning disabilities; investigating proposed structure of the classification; item-by-item evaluation of cross-cultural applicability; data on the boundaries of the classification system.

The CAR research was conducted at 20^1 sites in a total of 16 nations. Table 2 describes the number of informants represented in the data collected by all sites.

Table 2. Numbers of informants or data collection and reporting sessions

Method	Total N Numbers of participating centres
Translation and linguistic analysis	12 (3 used original English version)
Pile sorting	450 informants at 19 centres
Concept mapping	441 informants at 18 centres

Item and classification results

The CAR effort was highly successful, resulting in the direct modification of a number of items in ICIDH-2. The CAR data also provided invaluable direction for the development of epidemiological and other assessment instruments being developed in parallel to ICIDH-2. The data will be presented first by the specific data collection method used, followed by triangulated summary data.

Linguistic analysis

The majority of the key ICIDH-2 items were easily transferable from culture to culture and language to language. There are, however, some problematic concepts in ICIDH-2 that exhibit one or more of six types of primary linguistic incompatibility. These incompatibility problems can be grouped by the following categories.

Category 1: Concepts that were difficult or impossible to translate into one of the CAR study languages
Some ICIDH-2 terms and concepts were difficult or impossible to translate, because there was no equivalent term or cultural concept in the local

---

[1] The centres which completed all six data collection tasks were three sites in India (Bangalore, Chennai, and Delhi), Japan, The Netherlands, Nigeria, Romania, and Tunisia. Tunisia was responsible for data collection in Egypt, so there was no separate centre narrative for Egypt. In the end, no data was collected from China. The centres which collected all of the data except the focus group data included Canada, Greece, Luxembourg, Spain, Turkey (with sites in Ankara, Istanbul, and Antalya), and the United Kingdom. The United States site (Flagstaff) did not collect key informant interview data or concept mapping data. The Cambodian site was a later addition to the field group and provided a centre description, key informant interviews, focus group data, and the revised item evaluation data set. The sites that collected focus group data included Cambodia, India (three sites), Japan, The Netherlands, Nigeria, Romania, Tunisia, and the United States (Flagstaff).

language. Table 3 shows examples of these types of ICIDH-2 concepts, the linguistic problem, and at least one language in which the condition occurred.

Table 3.   Examples of linguistic equivalency problems

Concept or phrase	Problem	Language
1. Affect	Does not translate	Hindi
2. Affect	No idiomatic equivalent	Kannada
3. Disablement	No generic term in Arabic	Arabic
4. Disablement	Cannot be used as umbrella term	Hindi
5. Executive function	Difficult to translate	Hindi, Tamil

Category 2: Concepts whose translation contained a narrowed connotation of the original term, changing the meaning of the original in one of the CAR study languages.

A number of ICIDH-2 concepts could be translated into a participating centre language, but the translation left out connotations that were present in the original term. This makes the concepts only partially equivalent. In some cases, the problem could be overcome by adding additional words or phrases to expand the concept. In other cases, no satisfactory solution was found for the shift in meaning. This could lead to a problem in interpreting data between two centres, if the concepts were embedded in survey questions or coding of classification items. Table 4 provides examples of concepts and words that typify this condition.

Table 4. Examples of concepts and terms with partial equivalency with English

Concept or phrase	Problem	Language
1. Affect	Refers only to emotional state	Tamil
2. Affect	Partial overlap with sentiment	Romanian
3. Handling everyday physical environment	Partial overlap, but primary meaning is temperature, humidity (domestic environment better)	Romanian
4. Well being	Attached to life, not health	Arabic

Category 3: Concepts the translation of which contained an elaborated set of connotations different from the original term, changing its meaning in one of the CAR study languages.

A number of ICIDH-2 concepts could be translated into a participating centre language, but the translated term had a larger range of connotations than the original term. This makes the concepts only partially equivalent. In some cases, the problem could be overcome by adding additional words or phrases to narrow the concept. In other cases, no satisfactory solution was found for the shift in meaning. Table 5 provides examples of concepts and words that exemplify this condition.

Table 5. Examples of concepts and terms with partial equivalency or with additional multiple connotations that interfere with equivalency

Concept or phrase	Problem	Language
1. Affect	Multiple meanings beyond the English	Dutch
2. Function	Translates as act, work, action	Kannada

Category 4: Distinct concepts in the English of ICIDH-2 that translate into a single term when translated into one of the CAR study languages.

There were a number of concepts that identify distinctly different meanings in English, but lose those distinctions when translated into one of the languages of the CAR centres. If these concepts are used in the classification system to distinguish different conditions, functions, processes or elements of the classification system, then the loss of distinction through overlap has the potential for creating confusion between supposedly distinct categories when the classification system is used in other cultures. Examples of the concepts and phrases which included this type of linguistic problem are identified in Table 6.

Table 6. Concepts and terms that merged during translation-back translation

Concept or phrase	Problem	Language
1. Disease	Disease, illness, sickness are interchangeable	Hindi
2. Disease	Disease and illness are interchangeable	Romanian
3. Disorder	Feeling ill, not healthy, illness	Kannada
4. Disorder	Disease and disorder synonymous	Tamil
5. Disorder	Disease and disorder translate to same term	Hindi

Category 5: Cross-culturally inapplicable definitions or examples.

A number of items could be conceptually transferred to the other languages through translation, but the definitions or examples that were used to explain the item contained elements that were cross-culturally inappropriate. There were also a few terms and definitions that were inappropriate for use in one or more cultural contexts, because of local cultural values. These conditions were identified in the linguistic analysis at the various sites. The following are examples of items or contextual conditions that caused problems in translating the definitions of the ICIDH-2 items:

Keeping appropriate physical contact and maintenance of social space
Problems with this item arose at both the Kannada (Bangalore) and Tamil (Chennai) centres in India. The idea of social space is difficult to translate in both languages, and the conventions for touching or not touching are very different from European cultures. The local investigators recommended changes in the original English, to make the examples more culturally appropriate.

Dating and forming relationships
Dating is predominantly a European and North American concept and is a very uncommon activity in a number of cultures, especially those where most marriages are still arranged. Several different centres in the Middle East and Asia pointed out that the concept is not relevant in some cultures or local ethnic groups, and should be changed either to be more generic (to include arranged marriages, or to include family-sponsored courting systems), or be presented as an optional category.

Overview of the results of the linguistic analysis

The data set for the terms that were identified by various centres as raising one of these types of linguistic issues are set out in List A and List B found in Appendix A of Chapter 3. List A is a terminology and concept list containing all potentially problematic terms in the introduction and explanatory sections of the ICIDH-2 classification. These terms were identified during the pilot study (described in Chapter 3) as being especially difficult to translate conceptually in at least two languages. Additional terms were added when they were discovered in the translation phase of the project to be problematic. List B is a list of terms (and accompanying definitions) that were derived from the key two-digit coding level item list for ICIDH-2. Again, the terms in the list are primarily the ones shown by the pilot study to be problematic. A few were added during the translation phase of the overall CAR project.

When the lists of problematic concepts from each of these categories were compared, it was found that several ICIDH-2 concepts and terms exhibited problems in more than one category. The problem concepts are summarized in Table 7.

These problem items provided an excellent starting point for recommending changes in the English version of ICIDH-2. Others present problems in a single language, and will need to be addressed in that language only. The options are to use a borrowed term, for concepts that do not exist in the language, but can be borrowed from another language; to add descriptive phrases or modifications to an existing term that partially captures the meaning in the original; or to combine existing words into unusual new combinations that can be used to explain the concepts in the classification. In a few cases, parts of the classification system may not be culturally applicable in a small number of cultures. Those specific items may need to be ignored in those cultures. It will be important to note those areas of incompatibility and to deal with them appropriately during the development of instruments for epidemiological and policy purposes.

Table 7.   Identification of multi-site cross problems with individual terms, List A

Term or concept	Type of linguistic problem
1. Affect	Difficult to translate (Hindi, Kannada); multiple or reduced meaning (Tamil, Dutch, Romanian)
2. Community	Multiple or reduced meaning, overlap on translation (Dutch, Tamil)
3. Disability	Difficult to translate, multiple or reduced meaning (Dutch, Tamil)
4. Disablement	Difficult to translate in multiple languages (Arabic, Hindi); translated English terms overlap (Tamil)
5. Disease	Translated English terms overlap (Romanian, Hindi)
6. Disorder	Translated English terms overlap (Hindi, Kannada)
7. Executive functions	Difficult to translate (Hindi, Tamil)
8. Function	Multiple or reduced meaning (Kannada, Romanian); difficult to translate, overlap on translation (Hindi, Tamil)
9. Handling everyday environment	Multiple or reduced meaning (Hindi, Romanian)
10. Impairment	Difficult to translate (Tamil); multiple or reduced meaning (Arabic)
11. Integrity	Multiple or reduced meaning (Kannada, Tamil)
12. Non-verbal	Multiple or reduced meaning (Hindi, Kannada, Tamil)
13. Quality of life	Multiple or reduced meaning, overlap on translation (Hindi, Tamil)
14. Well-being	Multiple or reduced meaning (Arabic, Tamil)

Pile sort data analyses

Quantitative results

The pile sort data for the CAR project constitute the largest effort to collect cross-cultural pile sort data yet published. Each centre provided pile sort data from a selected group of respondents, as well as concept mapping data either

from the same respondents or from individuals in the same respondent categories. This data collection process allowed for concept comparison both within
and between cultural groups. It allowed the data to be compared from country
to country, language group to language group and between key social positions
across cultures (health providers compared with lay individuals, and so on).

The raw data for each respondent were typed as ASCII files and imported
into a computer program, ANTHROPAC 3.0 (Borgatti 1996). The program
contains a data conversion routine that transforms raw pile sort data into an
item-by-item similarities matrix. The matrix data were then analyzed using
multivariate statistics. One of the analytical processes was to create a Johnson's
hierarchical cluster analysis dendrogram of pile sort data (Johnson 1990),
and another process was a correlational analysis algorithm (Qualitative Analysis Programme, QAP) that allowed us to compare the classification solutions
between cultures and groups. The cluster analysis solution for the total data
set was created using the Johnson's hierarchical algorithm in ANTHROPAC.
The resulting data points and icicle plots were evaluated for cut points, both
through visual inspection and by removing random sets of informants from
the data set, to identify stable clusters. A stable grouping of 12 clusters of
items was identified.

This raw data set resulted in the identification of the following stable
clusters:

Cluster 1: Items relating to participation in community life
community
- Civic and community life
- Citizenship responsibilities
- Following (showing interest in) events that take place outside of the direct
  environment
- Leisure
- Cultural activities
- Religious activities

Cluster 2: Interaction with other persons
- Keeping appropriate physical contact, and maintenance of social space
- Interacting with an equal, co-worker, peer
- Showing tolerance in relationships
- Managing close personal relationships
- Interpersonal and social relationships

- Managing relationships with friends
- People sharing living space
- Keeping rules, abiding by decisions

Cluster 3: Sexual activities
- Sexual functions
- Dating and forming a sexual relationship
- Performing consensual sexual acts

Cluster 4: Taking care of work and economic responsibilities
- Economic self-sufficiency
- Activities related to fulfilling of financial obligations and services work
- Work acquisition and retention behaviours

Cluster 5: Daily living activities (two sub-cluster)
- Maintaining physical environment
- Handling everyday physical environment

- Taking care of ones health
- Dressing
- Self care
- Keeping self clean and appropriately groomed
- Washing oneself
- Eating and drinking
- Cooking, baking, frying solid
- Planning and organizing meals
- Taking care of meals
- Procurement and care of necessities
- Taking care of pets and domestic animals
- Taking care of household or family members
- Organizing daily routine
- Monitoring and evaluating of performance of activities and tasks

Cluster 6: Mobility
- Motor coordination

- Mobility
- Transferring oneself
- Moving around
- Changing a body position
- Maintaining a body position
- Handling technical devices, aids for locomotion
- Handling body attached technical aids
- Using public transport

Cluster 7: Communication
- Understanding specific signs
- Use of humour
- Following written instructions
- Following verbal instructions
- Visual sensory perceptions
- Using special means of communication
- Use of communication devices
- Non-verbal means of communication
- Written communication
- Communication activities
- Communication content
- Conversation processes and structure
- Responding to conversational cues

Cluster 8: Learning activities (two sub-clusters)
- Problem solving
- Arithmetic activities
- Acquiring and applying knowledge
- Abilities related to learning
- Study behaviours
- Education

Cluster 9: Sensory activities
- Experience of pain

- Seeing
- Visual sensory functions
- Hearing functions
- Hearing

Cluster 10: Attention, thought, and memory
- Thought, abstraction, judgement, and related executive functions
- Intellectual development and function
- Recognizing directions in space and time
- Orientation
- Perception
- Memory
- Attention
- Consciousness
- Recognizing
- Psychomotor activity

Cluster 11: Emotionally related activities
- Energy and drive
- Performing an activity for an extended period
- Managing general psychological demands
- Expressing empathy
- Temperament and personality
- Affect
- Managing personal behaviour

Cluster 12: Responding to danger
- Managing a dangerous environment
- Responding to dangers

These data indicate that the structure of the classification system, as a whole, represents a cross-culturally stable organization of the relationships among these items, when viewed within a cross-cultural context. While some individual items are not yet cross-culturally applicable, or stable, the overall structure of the classification (i.e., the organization of the items into specific clusters within the classification) meets the needs and represents the composite viewpoint of both health professionals and individuals directly affected by disabilities across very diverse cultures, language groups, and levels of economic development at the participating centres.

The overall stability of the cluster pattern was checked by randomly removing 30% of the informant responses from the total data set, and then both regenerating the cluster solution with the modified data set and comparing the modified data set with the total data set, utilizing the QAP routine in ANTHROPAC. Second, each separate site data set was compared to the total data set, utilizing the QAP routine. The finding was that the cluster solutions demonstrate a high level of stability within and between or across sites.

The following conditions apply to the overall data cluster solution. The clusters correspond closely to many of the chapters of the ICIDH-2 classification. This indicates that the classification has significant cross-cultural stability in its structure, since the piles that created these clusters were unconstrained (i.e. they were not created using cues about how to cluster them). The items highlighted by asterisks are items that are very stable cross-culturally, and are likely to be the best points for creating stable questions for cross-cultural questionnaires. The weakest items (those that are only loosely tied to a specific cluster) are the items that have the least cross-cultural consensus about their placement. This indicates some form of cross-cultural ambiguity that needs to be resolved by changing the item, or defining it more clearly.

The cross-culturally problematic phrases and concepts identified by the pile sort process were those that individual respondents had significant amounts of difficulty in placing within the classification system. Each of these items contains one or more conceptual elements that make them difficult to translate and to be understood in several cultures, or elements that cannot be easily associated with the other items in the classification system, because of extreme cross-cultural variation in the activity, or in the assumptions attached to the condition. These items have been examined for either significant revision or removal from the concepts used in ICIDH-2.

The problematic items include: "using public transportation," "problem solving," "understanding specific signs," "psychomotor activity," "energy and drive," "managing personal behaviour." Some items, such as "religious activities" and "pain," were often placed in a separate, single-item category. Others, as well as items, such as "following events that take place outside the direct environment" were often consistently placed in two or more clusters. Several items were not understood cross-culturally, such as "sharing living space" or "use of humour." Finally, there were a number of concepts and phrases that could be classified within clusters, but showed only very marginal association with the clusters.

Qualitative analysis of pile sort data

The pile sort data were analyzed by qualitative methods as well as the quantitative approach described above. As a second test for the presence or absence of cross-culturally ambiguous items, those that individuals had difficulty in placing in any specific pile were analyzed on the basis of the information given in the "reasons for pile sort and pile label" cards accompanying each pile.

The pile sort technique nearly always produces a "residual or miscellaneous" category as part of the classification process. These items can be separately identified and interpreted as items problematic for the classification system as a whole. An analysis of these items for the CAR study demonstrated two types of difficulty for the classification: within culture ambiguity and cross-cultural ambiguity. Some items were found to be hard to associate with other items by the people doing the pile sorting at certain sites, but not at others. These, and a second set of items that were identified in "miscellaneous" piles in multiple cultures, are being utilized to target domains for change in the revision process. These items provide a cross-check with the data derived from the mathematical models of the pile sorts, and from the statistical analysis of the concept mapping data analysis conducted for the CAR study. The results confirmed that the items listed above as problematic match those that were ambiguous for the pile sorting, and those that occasioned the most cross-cultural difficulties in the concept mapping exercise.

The pile sort technique is ideal for comparing cross-cultural views on classification systems. The items that show a clear cross-cultural stability and high saliency in the cluster analysis may be strong candidates for anchors for the development of instruments to assess the ICIDH-2 domains, or to use in a short form for assessment of the population. Items for the ICIDH-2 epidemiological and assessment instruments have subsequently been drawn from items that demonstrate high stability in the pile sort cluster analysis. Those items that show the least stability in the pile sort analysis were therefore poor choices as core items for instrument development. The underlying dimensions demonstrated by the multi-dimensional scaling of the pile sort data indicate that a) the overall structure of the classification includes the concept of simple to complex domains, based on complexity of task ; and b) the domains recommended for instrument development capture the majority of the underlying principles embedded in the classification system

Concept mapping results

The concept mapping analysis identified a list of items that were problematic on any of the 10 questions asked about (see Chapter 3 for details): clarity of the item; clarity of the underlying concept; usability of the item for the culture; usability of the item for all age groups; usability of the item for both sexes; usability of the item for all socioeconomic groups; usability of the item for ethnic and minority groups; cultural sensitivity of items; classification of the items into the levels of impairment, activity, or participation; and importance of the item for ICIDH-2 as a whole.

Table 8 gives examples of items that showed problems either in clarity of the item or its definition. All items that caused problems for at least 20% of the respondents are listed in order from the most problematic to the least problematic.

Table 8. Items and definitions with most problematic scores in the concept mapping

Item name (classification)	Problems %	
	Item	Definition
Community (Participation)	28.6	21.9
Thought, abstraction, judgement, and related Executive functions (Impairment)	24.3	21.9
Orientation (Impairment)	21.4	9.4
Performing an activity for an extended period (psychological endurance) (Activity)	21.1	15.1
Affect (Impairment)	20.7	12.5
Managing general psychological demands (Activity)	20.6	13.9
Keeping appropriate physical contact, and maintenance of social space (Activity)	20.5	12.0

Note: Percentages of problems indicate proportion of respondents who had problems with either the clarity of the item or the clarity of the concept or definition.

Overall, the concept mapping showed a high degree of cross-cultural compatibility of the items in the draft revision of ICIDH-2. This can be seen from the fact that only a very small proportion of the items tested caused problems for more than 20% of the respondents with clarity of either the item or the concept (see Table 8 above). Some items, however, required reconceptualization.

The classification of items into the three levels – Impairments, Activities, and Participation – was not sufficiently clear to all participants: 54.2% of the participant classifications did not correspond to the actual classification in ICIDH-2. As a result, the introduction of the subsequent Beta-2 draft of ICIDH-2 was amended to better explain the new structure and its underlying assumptions. The general results of the concept mapping by disability dimension of ICIDH-2 are summarized in Table 9.

Overall, the Participation disability dimension showed the most problems, especially with regard to usefulness of the items for different subgroups in a culture (age groups, gender, social group, ethnic or minority groups). On the other hand, the Participation items were clearest in terms of their classification within ICIDH-2 – i.e., people made fewer errors in classifying them into Participation.

Table 9. Descriptive results of concept mapping by ICIDH-2-level

	Impairments	Activies	Participation
Clarity of item (% problems)	14.8	12.6	15.0
Clarity of definition (% problems)	12.0	9.6	14.0
Usable in culture (% no)	5.3	5.6	7.1
Usable for all age groups (% no)	8.5	15.0	19.9
Usable for both gender (% no)	3.1	5.8	8.4
Usable for all social economic groups (% no) Usable for ethnic or minority groups (% no)	3.8	5.1	8.4
Culturally sensitive (%)	8.7	7.9	6.9
Misclassified (%)	58.7	55.5	34.4
Importance* Mean	2.4	2.4	2.41
Standard deviation	1.23	1.14	1.13

* (1=not important – 4=very important)

There was most variability between items with respect to questions about usefulness for all age groups and about taboo. Items that were judged to pose most problems with respect to application in all age groups (at least 25% of the sample indicated problems with usability in all age groups) were the following:

Economic self-sufficiency
Work
Activities related to fulfilling financial obligations and services
Cooking, baking, frying solids
Taking care of meals
Dating and forming relationships
Sexual functions
Performing consensual sexual acts

Not surprisingly, the last three items on this list were the only ones seen as prone to be culturally sensitive or taboo (again 25% was taken as the cut-off point).

Overall there was some cultural variability as the results in the country reports suggest (see Chapter 19 above). An important result of the concept mapping analysis was that the dimensions represented by the 10 questions asked were not independent and could be reduced to five dimensions. This was shown by factor analytic techniques taking into account that the underlying data structure was only ordinal (i.e., problem vs. no problem; see Jöreskog 1979). The five dimensions become possible because the questions on item and concept clarity loaded on one factor (with factor loadings of 1.0 and 0.86 respectively), all the usability items loaded on a second factor (useful in culture 0.81; useful in all age groups 0.77; useful in both genders 0.83; useful in all socioeconomic groups 1.0; useful in ethnic/minority groups 0.91), and the other items had dimensions (factors) of their own. The emerging factors correlate only to a small degree with each other (between 0.01 and 0.44), with an average correlation of 0.15 (detailed results of the confirmatory factor analysis are available from the first author). As a result, the subsequent field test used only five dimensions in the concept mapping exercise, thus reducing the workload by 50%.

Conclusion

A mixture of quantitative and qualitative techniques was used to study the cross-cultural applicability of the items and concepts in ICIDH-2. A formal translation/back-translation protocol was used to establish equivalences of linguistic terms. Pile sorting and concept mapping identified problems with different structures in different cultures as well as problematic items and concepts. The results of these methods converged to a considerable degree and triangulation was used to identify the most problematic items and concepts. These were changed for the new ICIDH-2 field test version. Moreover, it was found that the classification of items into the three dimensions of disability, namely Impairments, Activities, and Participation was not sufficiently clear to all participants. As a result, the new structure of ICIDH-2 and its underlying assumptions had to be better explained in the introduction of the next, Beta-2, version of ICIDH-2. Finally, the results were used to improve the methodology of the subsequent field tests.

Chapter 21
Summary and Conclusions

*T.B. Üstün, S. Chatterji, J.E. Bickenbach, R. T. Trotter II, R. Room,
J. Rehm, and S. Saxena**

The effectiveness of the CAR methodological suite

The CAR suite of methods, by combining the strengths of both qualitative
and quantitative research, provided excellent and extensive information to
guide the ICIDH-2 revision. At the same time, these methods allow the accommodation of a substantial degree of cross-cultural variation that would
otherwise hinder the development of a universal language. The methods were
chosen to complement each other, and this combination met the need for
triangulation, that is, the need to substantiate the findings by means of multiple data collection procedures. This combination of methods also helped to
satisfy the statistical requirements of reliability and validity. In addition, each
of the methods on its own produced significant results.

Linguistic analysis

The concept mapping and linguistic evaluation exercises were intended to
examine the effectiveness of the conceptual transfer that elements of a classification must undergo in order to meet the minimum requirements for a
truly universal language. In the past, the standard procedure for making a
document cross-culturally applicable has been to run it through a translation
and back-translation process, in order to identify any problems with lan-

---
* WHO, Assessment, Classification and Epidemiology Group, Geneva, Switzerland (Üstün, Chatterji,
Saxena); Department of Philosophy, Queen's University, Kingston, Ontario, Canada (Bickenbach);
Department of Anthropology, Northern Arizona University, Flagstaff, Arizona, USA (Trotter); Centre
for Addiction and Mental Health, Addition Research Foundation Division, Toronto, Ontario, Canada
(Room, Rehm).

guage. However, this process has been shown to be only partially effective. As a result, the CAR study incorporated an expanded translation and linguistic analysis protocol.

First, the translation was accompanied by a concept mapping and linguistic problem reporting process that not only identified problems in translating words from English into other languages, but showed problems of ambiguity in the original language as well. This allowed the simultaneous improvement of the classification in the original language and in the target language. Second, the linguistic analysis protocol used an innovative approach in providing, for a selected list of the terms, sentences in English that illustrated the nuances and connotations of the terms. This enabled translators to capture the intended use of the terms without necessarily being restricted by the back translation process.

The linguistic protocol identified problems at the level of terms in the classification (which were then appropriately modified or clarified), at the level of concepts (leading to the modification of definitions and structural relationships), and at the theoretical level (suggesting improvements in the rationale and structure of the classification as a whole). For example, most sites reported problems with translation of the term "disablement" to encompass the negative aspects of the three dimensions of functioning (namely, impairments, activity limitations and participation restrictions). As a result, the term was replaced with a more common term – "disability" – as the new umbrella term.

It is gratifying to note that fewer than 10% of the elements were considered problematic. It is, however, quite clear that in people's minds disability is a unitary experience often difficult to separate into impairments, activity limitations and participation restrictions. Although items belonging to the last category are clearly distinguished from the other two, they were found to present the greatest difficulty in cross-cultural application.

Pile sorting

The stability of items and their conceptual boundaries were explored by means of the pile sorting exercise. This is a method used in cognitive anthropology, where it is designed to explore the relationship of items in a cultural domain, in this case, the relationships of items in a classification of disabilities.

The CAR study was able to collect samples of the ways in which individuals from many different cultures would create a natural or indigenous classification out of the two-digit items in the ICIDH-2 classification, without any necessary reference to the existing classification. These samples showed how the items would be clustered into groups that were meaningful within a particular culture. We were then able to provide three types of information for the revision process. First, it was clear that there was a core set of concepts (items and definitions) that were very stable across cultures. These items form the conceptual and practical core of the ICIDH-2 classification and their stability provides strong evidence that the structure of the classification is not only theoretically viable, but is empirically validated across multiple languages and cultures. Second, the process allowed each language and culture group potentially to identify the items and concepts that differed from the global core in their language and culture. This information is valuable for local translation, and construction of a defensible classification that is true to the original. Third, the process identified problematic items that needed to be addressed in the original classification, since there were far too many cross-cultural differences in the ways they were placed in the classification in multiple languages and cultures.

There are several examples of changes made to the classification as a result of the findings from the pile sorting, especially when these results were combined with the linguistic analysis and the concept mapping results. For example, terms such as "executive function" as a technical term were not understood, and the term "environment" raised difficulties in several languages.

Concept mapping

The concept mapping process was intended as a structured and quantitative supplement to focus groups as a method for exploring items within the classification across several dimensions. It provided highly specific data at the item and definition level of the classification. However, the study design was too ambitious and so resulted in a heavy burden on respondents. The information on individual items was valuable, but the number of questions asked, the repetitive nature of the exercise, and the number of individuals who indicated that they had trouble completing the exercise reduced the usefulness of the data somewhat. The problem items identified in this process were very similar to those identified by the pile sort and the linguistic analysis. Concept mapping allowed the exact nature of the problem to be explored (whether, for example, it was an issue of cultural taboo or insensitivity to age, gender, and so on). However, there should have been fewer than 10 questions asked for the 90 items, and the structure of the questions should have been improved. This was taken into account in the subsequent ICIDH-2 field trials, with much improved results.

Despite these problems, the information was extremely valuable for the revision process and to help the centres learn about the cross-cultural issues in the classification. Some of the terms that were found to be culturally sensitive at a number of sites were not used as key terms in the classification and others that were unclear were defined more explicitly to increase their ability to be understood.

Key informant interviews

The key informant interview procedure is standard, and has been used many times for this type of purpose (Trotter & Schenshul 1998; Bernard 1998). Traditionally, key informant interviews have relied on qualitative interpretations of verbatim records of such interview material. In this case it included qualitative open-ended questions supplemented by quantitative exercises that have proven very valuable. These interviews give us important evidence about the general level of social support for disabled persons, the governmental and nongovernmental responsibilities for assistance, and the relative rankings of disabilities in terms of their social impact within the culture. The results of this study were especially valuable because of the wide cross-section of key informants included. All of this information was used for expanding and revising the evolving disability paradigm embedded in ICIDH-2. The information was also useful in developing the conceptual framework for the ICIDH-2 based disability assessment instrument (WHODAS-II), and will be helpful in the future to further develop the notion of burden of disease and use of disability-adjusted life years (DALYs) as a summary health measure (Murray & Lopez 1996).

Focus groups

The focus groups provided some valuable information for the CAR study, especially in the description of cultural variability of stigma, information about assistance models, and both familial and societal attitudes and responses to disabling conditions. Also explored was the issue of the lack of parity in the treatment, both by governments and by society at large, of people with physical disabilities as compared with those with mental disabilities. The method was thus valuable for the overall revision process. Moreover, all centres commented that the information produced by this method was very valuable. It was almost universally remarked that focus groups provided the centre researchers with important information about disabilities in their cultures and that they had not been exposed to at this level of detailed information in the past. The information helped the centres to acquire different viewpoints about disabilities, as well as a better understanding of the social processes that surround disabling conditions.

In conclusion, all of these qualitative methods, separately and in combination, did the job they were designed to do. In many instances, too, substantial new information about disabilities was acquired by the centres that participated in the study. We certainly recommend that the methods be used together, in a coordinated manner, for future cross-cultural applicability studies.

Principal results

The meaning of disability

One of the important findings of the CAR study is the confirmation that disability has multiple meanings that must be accommodated in a classification, and that no one meaning holds the key to the future of disability policy. The study incorporated processes (both data collection and revision strategies) that included multiple simultaneous viewpoints from disability researchers, policy-makers, persons with disabilities, care-givers, and the general public. This created a process that aimed at achieving the right balance of legitimate viewpoints, which, though difficult to carry out, greatly strengthened the outcome.

In spite of the rich diversity of viewpoints expressed and the explicit recognition of differences in the way disability issues are construed the world over, it was also gratifying to note the commonalities across the centres. Uniformly, respondents pointed out the stigma associated with disability, the lack of parity between mental health, alcohol and substance use and physical health conditions, and the role of physical and attitudinal barriers in the construction of disability. That disability needs to be understood as a social as well as a medical construct was amply highlighted. It was also clear that across the world disability is understood as an experience that affects the body and mind, the person as a whole and societal interaction in general. This conception of disability is uniform across centres, although respondents were not always sure how to deal with "invisible" disabilities (such as some forms of cognitive impairments) or those for which in some way the person is held responsible.

The role of social attitudes in the disablement process

The CAR data lead to a number of insights into the role of social attitudes towards disabilities. In each society, social attitudes are imbedded in the accommodation and compensation systems that were described by the CAR centres. Attitudes differed according to cultural assumptions about the responsibility of persons with disabilities for both the cause and the accommodation of the disability.

In some cases, there are competing or conflicting cultural views about causation. In some cultures, a person is treated more sympathetically, and provided with more public support for accommodation, when the disability is the result of a birth defect or an accident than if there are other causes. In these cultures, the condition is seen as not being the fault of the individual or his or her family, and therefore deserving social compensation or accommodation. In a very few cultures, both physical and mental health problems are seen in this light, and are treated with something close to parity. However, the opposite view prevails in a large number of cultures. Both accidents of birth and accidental physical injury are seen as linked to prior or current social and spiritual transgressions on the part of either the individual or the individual's family. In these cultures, the family is seen as being at fault and the societal values do not support governmental or societal accommodation of the disability. This complicates the stance of etiological neutrality in ICIDH-2, and places these societies in conflict with cultural norms that are aggressively attempting to destigmatize disabilities, and to achieve parity between mental and physical health conditions. This is a key cultural diversity issue raised by the CAR study and one that will need significant attention in the future.

Etiological neutrality

The model of disability in ICIDH-2 classifies dimensions of disability independently of their causal or etiological background. This means, in part, that no assumption is made within the classification of the likely or necessary causes of any activity limitation or participation restriction. Etiological neutrality, as this assumption is called, ensures that ICIDH-2 can be used by many and diverse users without committing them to any particular theory about the causes of disability. The CAR study results clearly support the need for etiological neutrality in the overall classification, while at the same time indicating that the lack of etiological neutrality in the cultural views of disabilities around the world has significant social impacts.

Parity

There are two important findings in the CAR data relating to parity. First, it is clear that mental health conditions, and the social behaviour that accompanies those conditions, is far more threatening to society at large than most physical health conditions. This threat is caused by a deviation from expected social interactions, and an inability to predict social responses at work, in public, and to a lesser extent at home. The effect of this threat is expressed in lack of social support for alcohol- and drug-related disabilities (since these are perceived to be self-inflicted), and for the lack of parity in programmes for disabilities associated with mental health conditions compared with common physical impairments (for example, blindness, deafness, or paraplegia). While ICIDH-2 is designed to accommodate the activity limitations produced by disabilities associated with either mental or physical health conditions, most societies are not yet ready to relinquish differential treatment of the consequences of the two different conditions. This disparity must be taken into account when using ICIDH-2 internationally.

A second finding is that there are a number of societies in which the issue of parity between physical and mental impairments is effectively a moot point at this time. These are cultures in which all forms of disability are so highly stigmatized that it is irrelevant to try to make distinctions between the causal factors. In these cases, the social stigma and consequences of disabilities become of prime importance for addressing the needs of disabled persons in the society, and the lack of parity then becomes a secondary factor.

Ranking the severity of disabilities

Concerns are often raised about whether people's perceptions of the severity of a disabling condition in comparison to another are uniform across settings and populations. When the key informants in this study were asked to conduct ratings on the disabling effects of different health conditions, it was understood that the diversity of informants, sites, languages, and cultures would allow us to develop a sense of whether these conditions are rated similarly or differently across cultures and informant groups.

Since the key informants were also asked about social disapproval and stigma, it was possible to consider the extent to which the ranking of severity of a disabling condition was a function of the stigma or disapproval in society. The study results showed consistently that higher stigma was associated with higher disability ratings. However, stigma was not the major determinant of the ranking.

In fact, it is worthy of note that although there is some variation in ranking by key informants of the disabling effect of health conditions, such rankings are overall relatively stable across countries and informant groups. In the eyes of the respondents the relative burden of different health conditions in terms of disabilities was fairly similar across the world. The results also indicate, however, that there are systematic cultural differences, as well as differences between informant groups. These differences are large enough to need to be further explored in a systematic way, with a triangulation of in-depth qualitative and quantitative methods.

The actual burden of disability is affected by the physical and social environment that creates the context in which the individual lives. For example, the burden of disability for persons with paraplegia depends on the available assistive devices (wheelchairs, adapted cars, adapted workplaces) and on the social support available. This would lead one to believe that the weight that people ascribe to different conditions will vary widely across settings. Clearly, there are differences between countries in terms of services and attitudes, and these differences should be reflected in different disability weights attached to certain health conditions. This may in fact happen when valuation of health states includes the assessment of several other parameters that influence the health experience.

The most variable condition in our sample is HIV infection, which was ranked from the most disabling of all health conditions presented in Egypt and Tunisia to the third least disabling condition in Luxembourg. The differences expressed by expert groups are less dramatic but still important. Doubtless, the differential availability of expensive treatment or the varying degree of stigma may contribute to these quite different judgements.

In general, physical conditions are ranked more uniformly and universally compared to mental conditions across countries. Physical conditions such as quadriplegia and vitiligo are almost always considered the most and the least disabling respectively, but mental health conditions often fall in the intermediate range and show the most variation across centres. This is not true, though, when comparisons are made across persons who either have the health condition themselves or care for someone with such a condition. The lived experience with a disabling health condition seems to override other determinants of the value attached to disability. In other words, though aggregated responses across countries seem to show a common pattern, individual health experiences influence the judgements of severity of health states rather differently. These results have important consequences for the assignment of disability weights for the calculation of burden of disease using the DALYs measure (see Üstün et al. 1999).

Social disapproval and stigma

The extensive data obtained from the key informants in this study reveal some clear messages. Drug- and alcohol-related conditions are always more stigmatized than mental disorders, and these are in turn are more stigmatised than physical disorders. Disabilities associated with these conditions also meet with social disapproval in the same order. Predictably, while respondents seem to consider conditions for which the individual is somehow seen as responsible (such as drug and alcohol disorders) as the most stigmatizing, they are willing to consider environmental factors that may have brought on the disability to be mitigating. Issues raised by genetic causes of disability, and whether or not they are present at birth, are complex and viewed differently in societies where cultural beliefs such as the doctrine of karma, prevail. There is no doubt, in general, that social attitudes and moral values are key factors in determining how people across the world view disabilities.

Cultural diversity versus universality in ICIDH-2

Qualitative research provides us with an understanding of the meaning that people attach to different concepts. It gives us insights into how these concepts "live" for the subjects of the research inquiry. To ensure that these insights are well grounded, researchers must allow concepts and theory to emerge from the data in order to develop hypotheses that can then be systematically tested (Strauss & Corbin 1994). Qualitative methods are best suited to the examination of complex situations where the exact nature of the relationships of several variables is not clearly understood. These methods allow for the generation of data for modelling the quantitative relationships between variables. The emergent results must be credible, transferable, confirmable and dependable (Hill 1991; Bernard 1998; Schensul & Le Compte 1999). The study findings should make evident sense.

The qualitative research used in the CAR study enabled us to recognize the differences as well as the commonalities across cultures in the perception and understanding of the disability construct. Cross-cultural research recognizes the "difference analysis" and the "search for similarities" as independent, and equally valuable, approaches that have different conceptual bases and methodological implications. Careful observation of a small subset of behaviours included under a hypothetical construct can capture the essential aspects of the construct, despite the wide variety of differences in manifest behaviour. This, then, is the rationale for finding a common set of variables that can form the basis for classification and measurement.

The underlying research agenda should attempt to find "equivalents" across cultures, while being aware of the factors that are responsible for the "bias" of differences. Results obtained in different cultures can then be used to evaluate the intercultural differences or else to assess the equivalent results across the different cultures.

Our results show that there is a considerable variation across our centres in terms of the language available to express disability constructs, the services for persons with disability, the attitudes towards and stigma surrounding disability, the acceptability in society of persons with disability, and the comparability of disability associated with physical and alcohol, drug and mental disorders.

In spite of these differences, however, some clear common themes have emerged. Disability is universally recognized as an aspect of the human health experience. Across cultures, the phenomena of disability are viewed as occurring at the level of the body functions or structures, at the level of the person in carrying out day-to-day activities, and as a direct result of barriers and hindrances that they encounter in their environment. Across the world, disabilities are stigmatized, though the extent and quality of this stigma varies and there is a clear bifurcation in attitudes about and services for people with physical health problems as opposed to those with alcohol, drug and mental disorders.

At the level of detail, the study makes it clear that, though living with a disability is a different experience across cultures, nonetheless there is agreement about which activities are essential to human functioning at the three levels. Across the centres, respondents tended to group together sets of activities that they felt were building blocks of human functioning. These range from interacting with one's environment, taking care of oneself, moving around and relating to others, to working and performing household activities and participating in a wide range of other social activities. Once again, though the manner of accomplishment of each of these vary, respondents uniformly recognize the importance of core human activities, from the relatively simple tasks of dressing and feeding oneself to more complex behaviours such as engaging in political activity or community events.

In the Introduction we described a fundamental dilemma for the revision of ICIDH-2, namely that, as an international classification providing a common language of disability, ICIDH-2 must offer a universal conceptual framework for disability across languages and cultures. Yet the experience of disability is, in some sense, unique to each individual, and anthropological and ethnographic research, including of course our own, suggests that this experience is in large part constructed from the cultural, linguistic and social environment in which each person lives. How can we create a universal language in the face of apparent cultural diversity? What has the CAR study to say about this dilemma?

If we recall the distinction earlier made between "weak" and "radical" relativism, the data presented in this volume make it abundantly clear that the radical position of complete and non-remediable incommensurability of the disability concept across cultures is radically mistaken. To be sure, the work reported here was preliminary, and can and should be extended to more countries and cultures, and involve more detailed features of ICIDH-2, both as a construct of disability and as a classification. Nonetheless, the results reported here make it apparent that the radical position is likely to be false or at least unjustifiable on the evidence.

It is understandable for researchers in the field to be impressed by the differences in their respondents' understanding of disability. They are, after all, highly attentive to differences. Similarities are often more difficult to detect. And fundamental similarities at the level of the construct itself – for example, that disability is a tripartite concept with clear differences between body, person and social levels – are even more difficult to identify. The CAR methodologies are, for reasons already explained, well suited to allow us to sift through the differences to identify the underlying similarities, without thereby falling into the opposite trap of discounting the differences as irrelevant or trivial.

For indeed the differences in cultural perceptions of disability are neither irrelevant nor trivial. The data presented in the previous two chapters make it clear that there are considerable cultural variations in perceptions of relative stigma, valuation, parity and underlying societal evaluation that are crucial to policy development. Refining these differences, and finding other, as yet undiscovered similarities, is work for the future. But we are in a position now to say with authority that the empirical evidence supports the possibility of a transcultural, common understanding of disability and, as well, an international common language of functioning and disability categories that can be used from country to country without surreptitiously imposing one cultural understanding on the rest of the world.

The CAR results, preliminary though they are, also indicate the importance of using state-of-the-art qualitative and quantitative research methodologies to acquire the empirical data needed to substantiate the many presuppositions about disability that one finds in the literature. In a recent note, Nora Groce claims that a cross-cultural perspective on disability shows that the disadvantages associated with disability are caused by the social environment (Groce 1999). Her claim may well be true. Unfortunately, we do not have the worldwide information to be sure *if* it is true, and more importantly, *how* in specific terms it is true. Without the data and the specifics, the claim takes on the appearance of a political slogan rather than an evidence-based claim.

What is ironic, though, is that often the scholars and researchers who firmly believe, to quote Groce again, that "the lives of individuals with disability are limited not so much by their specific type of disability as by the social interpretation of that disability" are radical relativists who refuse to grant the possibility of a universal disability construct, or the usefulness of an international classification such as ICIDH-2. This stance is, on the face of it, self-defeating, since the claim of environmental causation will remain a political slogan rather than a confirmed scientific hypothesis unless the measurement work can be done to demonstrate quantitatively how the environment causes the disadvantages of disability, and how we can change the environment to eliminate or alleviate these disadvantages.

The research challenge posed by the ICIDH-2 and related assessment instruments

Though the CAR study has demonstrated the feasibility of undertaking the mammoth exercise of developing a common language of disability within the wide diversity that exists cross- culturally, the task is far from complete. Certainly the results of the study indicate that technical language must be converted into simpler terminology and care will have to be taken to explain the theoretical and philosophical underpinnings to potential users. The challenge of making the classification useful for day-to-day applications, ranging from clinical uses to policy development, is being addressed by WHO through its strategies for implementing ICIDH-2 as well as associated assessment tools such as WHODAS II and the ICIDH-2 checklist.

Building a common language of disability that is not only cross-culturally valid but also lives up to its claim of being etiologically neutral in order to create parity across specific health conditions is, of course, a tall order. Ongoing field studies of ICIDH-2 and WHODAS II should provide empirical data on how these tools fulfil these goals. The need to establish workable thresholds for disability will continue to be addressed, as thresholds form the basis for many vital resource allocation decisions. Multidimensional assessment of disability, which distils several factors into a single metric, is also a challenge. The need to account for subjective perceptions of health states as well as individual and social valuations of them makes the situation even more complex and the task even more daunting.

The road ahead

In the future it is hoped that a true synthesis of the biological, psychological and social influences in the disability experience can be constructed and scientifically validated. This synthesis must be based on systematically collected evidence, not political rhetoric. ICIDH-2 offers a cross-cultural and international framework for collecting evidence that will assist researchers, policy-makers and advocates to understand more fully the impact of health conditions. The success of ICIDH-2 as the international common language for disability will be a fitting tribute to the cross-cultural applicability research described in this volume.

The road ahead

References

Adamczyk, P. (1994) Concept mapping: a multi-level and multi-purpose tool. *School Science Review,* 76, 275, 116.

Al-Kunifed, A. and Wandersee, J. H. (1990) One hundred references related to concept mapping. *Journal of Research in Science Teaching,* 27 (10), 1069.

American Psychiatric Association (1994) *Diagnostic and Statistical Manual of Mental Disorders* (4th edn) (DSM-IV). Washington, DC: APA.

Andrews, G., Sanderson, K, Beard, J. (1998) Burden of disease. Method of calculating disability from mental disorder. *British Journal of Psychiatry,* 173, 123–131.

Arabie P, Hubert, L.J, De Soete G. (eds.) (1997) *Clustering and Classification.* River Edge, NJ: World Scientific Publishing Co., Inc.

Asian Development Bank (1995) *First Round of National Socio-economic Survey in Cambodia.* In conjunction with Ministry of Planning, Phnom Penh.

Asian Development Bank (1997) *Second Round of National Socio-economic Survey in Cambodia.* In conjunction with Ministry of Planning, Phnom Penh.

Bakheit, A.M., Shanmugalingam, V. (1997) A study of the attitudes of a rural Indian community toward people with physical disabilities. *Clinical Rehabilitation,* 11, 329–334.

Basumallik, K.T., Bhattacharya, K.P. (1983) Views on mental health: A cross-cultural study. *Indian Journal of Clinical Psychology,* 10, 219–226.

Benedict, R. (1934) *Patterns of Culture.* New York: Houghton Mifflin.

Benedict, R. (1974) *The Chrysanthemum and the Sword: Patterns of Japanese Culture.* Tokyo: Charles E. Tuttle Co.

Bernard, H.R. (1995) *Research Methods in Cultural Anthropology.* Beverly Hills, CA: Sage Publications.

Berkasal, N. (1983) A controlled study about mental status and social adaptation of chronic schizophrenic and alcoholic patients. Dissertation thesis, Hacettepe University Psychiatry Clinic, Ankara.

Bice, T.W., Kalimo, E. (1971) Comparisons of health-related attitudes – a cross-national factor analytic study. *Social Science and Medicine,* 5, 283–318.

Bickenbach, J.E., Chatterji, S., Badley, E.M. et al. (1999) Models of disablement, universalism and the ICIDH. *Social Science and Medicine,* 48, 1173–87.

Borgatti, S. Anthropac. Greensboro, NC: Analytic Technologies 1996.

Cambodian Trust (1995) *Cambodian Children and Women with Artificial Limbs,* Children and Women's Prosthetic Outreach Programme Unit, Phnom Penh.

Central Bureau of Statistics (1999) *Statistisch Jaarboek 1998.* [Statistical Yearbook 1998.] Voorburg, Heerlen: Central Bureau of Statistics.

Central Bureau of Statistics/Netherlands Institute for Research on Social Welfare (1990) *Lichamelijke beperkingen bij de Nederlandse bevolking, 1986/1988.* [Physical disability in the population of the Netherlands, 1986/1988.] The Hague: Central Bureau of Statistics.

Chadda, R. (1996) Social support and psychosocial dysfunction in depression. *Indian Journal of Psychiatry,* 37(3), 119–123.

Chakrabarti, S., Lok Raj, Kulhara, P. et al. (1995) Comparison of the extent and pattern of family burden in affective disorders and schizophrenia. *Indian Journal of Psychiatry,* 37(3), 105–112.

Chamie, M. (1995) What does morbidity have to do with disability? *Disability and Rehabilitation,* 17, 323–327.

Coriel, J., Augustin, A., Holt, E. et al. (1992) Use of ethnographic research for instrument development in a case-control study of immunization use in Haiti. *International Journal of Epidemiology* (suppl. 2), s33–s37.

Courtright, P., Klungsoyr, P., Lewallen, S. et al. (1993) The epidemiology of blindness and visual loss in Hamar tribesmen of Ethiopia. The role of gender. *Tropical and Geographical Medicine,* 45, 168–170.

Coxon, T. (1999) *Sorting Data.* Beverly Hills, CA: Sage Publications

de Smidt, L.S. (1948) *Among the San Blas Indians of Panama.* New York, NY, Troy.

Devlieger, P., Piachaud, J., Leung, P. et al. (1994) Coping with epilepsy in Zimbabwe and the Midwest, USA. *International Journal of Rehabilitation Research,* 17, 251–264.

Domin, D.S. (1996) Comment: Concept mapping and representational systems. *Journal of Research in Science Teaching,* 33(8), 935.

Doyle, J., Wong, L.L. (1996) Mismatch between aspects of hearing impairment and hearing disability/handicap in adult/elderly Cantonese speakers: Some hypotheses concerning cultural and linguistic influences. *Journal of the American Academy of Audiology,* 7, 442–446.

Edmondson, K.M. (1995) Concept mapping for the development of medical curricula, *Journal of Research in Science Teaching,* 32: 7, 777.

Federal Ministry of Education (1981) Blue-print on education of the handicapped in Nigeria. In *The National Policy on Education.* Lagos: Federal Government Press.

Federal Office of Statistics (1996) *Socio-Economic Profile of Nigeria.* Lagos: Federal Government Press.

Fisher, A.G., Liu, Y., Velozo, C.A. et al. (1992) Cross-cultural assessment of process skills. *American Journal of Occupational Therapy,* 46, 876–885.

Fougeyrollas, P. (1995) Documenting environmental factors for preventing the handicap creation process: Quebec contributions relating to ICIDH and social participation of people with functional differences. *Disability and Rehabilitation,* 17, 145–153.

Gögüs, A. (1981) A controlled study on determination of social dysfunction in mental disorder. Dissertation thesis, Hacettepe University Psychiatry Clinic, Ankara.

Goodman, L. A. (1961) Snowball sampling. *Annals of Mathematical Statistics,* 32, 148–170.

Goodwin, C., Duranti, A. (1992) Rethinking Context: An Introduction. In Duranti, D. and Goodwin, C. (eds.) *Rethinking Context: Language as an Interactive Phenomenon.* Cambridge: Cambridge University Press, 1–42.

Groce, N. (1985) *Everyone Here Spoke Sign Language.* Cambridge, MA: Harvard University Press.

Groce, N. (1999) Disability in cross-cultural perspective: rethinking disability. *Lancet,* 354, 756–57

Halbertsma, J. (1995) The ICIDH: health problems in a medical and social perspective. *Disability and Rehabilitation,* 17, 128–134.

Handicap International (1997) *Cambodia 1996 Annual Report,* Phnom Penh.

Hill, C.E. (ed.) (1991) *Training Manual in Applied Medical Anthropology*. American Anthropological Association Special Publications No. 27. Washington, D.C., American Anthropological Association.

Ho, S.C., Woo, J., Lau, J. et al. (1995) Life satisfaction and associated factors in older Hong Kong Chinese. *Journal of the American Geriatric Society,* 43, 252–255.

Holmes, D., Splaine, M., Teresi, J. (1994) What makes special care special: concept mapping as a definition tool. *Alzheimer Disease and Associated Disorders.* 8 suppl, 41.

Ingstad, B., Whyte, S.R. (1995) *Disability and Culture.* Berkeley, CA: University of California Press.

Jitapunkul, S., Kamolratanakul, P., Ebrahim, S. (1994) The meaning of activities of daily living in a Thai elderly population: development of a new index. *Age and Ageing,* 23, 97–101.

Johnson, J., Boster, J.S., Holbert, D. (1989) Estimating relational attributes from snowball samples through simulation. *Social Networks* 11(4), 135–140.

Johnson J.C. (1990) *Selecting Ethnographic Informants.* Qualitative Research Methods (Vol. 22). Newbury Park, CA: Sage Publications.

Jöreskog, K.G. (1979) Basic ideas of factor and component analysis. In K.G. Jöreskog and Sörbom, D. (eds.) *Advances in Factor Analysis and Structural Equation Models.* Cambridge, MA: ABT, 5–20.

Kaplan C.D., Korf D., Sterk C. (1987) Temporal and social contexts of heroin-using populations. An illustration of the snowball sampling technique. *Journal of Nervous Mental Diseases* 175(9), 566–574.

Kaplan, I. (1995) Mental disorders and disability in a primary health care clinic in Semi-rural area. *Turkish Journal of Psychiatry,* 6(3), 169–179.

Kleinman, A. (1980) *Patients and Healers in the Context of Culture.* Berkeley, CA, University of California Press.

Klerk M.M.Y. de, Timmermans, J.M. (1998) *Rapportage gehandicapten 1997.* [Report on the handicapped 1997.] Rijswijk: Social and Cultural Planning Agency.

Krueger, R.A. (1994) *Focus Groups: A Practical Guide for Applied Research.* 2nd ed. Thousand Oaks, CA: Sage Publication.

Lane, S.D., Mikhail, B.I., Reizian, A. et al.. (1993) Sociocultural aspects of blindness in an Egyptian delta hamlet: Visual impairment vs. visual disability. *Medical Anthropology,* 15, 245–260.

Lord, C.G., Desforges, D. M., Fein, S. (1994) Typicality effect in attitudes toward social policies: A concept-mapping approach. *Journal of Personality and Social Psychology,* 66(4), 658.

Lucy, J. (1985) Whorf's view of the linguistic mediation of thought. In Mertz, E. and Parmentier, R. (eds.) *Semiotic Mediation.* Orlando, FL: Academic Press, 73–97.

Mercan, S., Ulug, B., Göğüs A. (1999) Cognitive functions and social disability in alcohol dependency. *Turkish Journal of Psychiatry,* 10(1), 3–12.

Ministry of Health (1995) *Population issues in the world and Turkey,* Ankara.

Ministry of Health and Welfare (1997) *Koseihakusyo.* Tokyo: Ministry of Health and Welfare.

Ministry of Health and Welfare (1999) *Social security policies in Japan.* Available on the internet at: http://www.mhw.go.jp/english/index.html (Sep. 1999).

Ministry of Social Affairs, Labour and Veteran Affairs (1995) *The situation of Disabled Persons in Cambodia.* Phnom Penh.

Morgan, D.L. (1988) Focus groups as qualitative research. Sage University Paper Series on Qualitative Research Methods (v. 16). Beverly Hills, CA, Sage Publications.

Murray, C.J.L., Lopez, A.D. (1996) *The Global Burden of Disease: a comprehensive assessment of mortality and disability from diseases, injuries, and risk factors in 1990 and projected to 2020.* Cambridge, MA: Harvard University Press.

Murray, C.J.L., Lopez, A.D. (1997) Global mortality, disability, and the contribution of risk factors. Global Burden of Disease study. *Lancet,* 349(9063), 1436–42.

Nunally, J.C. (1961) *Popular Conceptions of Mental Health: Their Development and Change.* New York: Holt, Reinhart & Winston.

Olfson, M., Fireman, B., Weissman M., et al. (1997) Mental disorders and disability among patients in a primary care group practice. *American Journal of Psychiatry,* 15, 12.

Opala, J., Boillot, F. (1996) Leprosy among the Limba: illness and healing in the context of world view. *Social Science and Medicine,* 42, 3–19.

Ormel, J., Van Korff, M., Üstün, B. et al. (1994) Common mental disorders and disability across cultures: results from the WHO collaborative study on psychological problems in general health care. *Journal of the American Medical Association,* 272, 1741–1748.

Patrick, J.H., Pruchno, R.A., Rose, M.S. (1998) Recruiting research participants: a comparison of the costs and effectiveness of five recruitment strategies, *Gerontologist* 38(3), 295–302.

Pezza, P.E. (1991) Value concept and value change theory in health education: a conceptual empirical methodological review. *Health Values,* 15(4), 3–12.

Pinker, S. (1994) *The Language Instinct.* New York, NY, William and Morrow.

Prabhu, G.G., Raguram, A., Verma, N. et al. (1984) Public attitudes towards mental illness: a review. *NIMHANS Journal,* 2, 1–14.

Quinn, N., Holland, D. (1987) *Cultural Models in Language and Thought.* New York, NY, Cambridge University Press.

Raymond, A.M. (1997) The use of concept mapping in qualitative research: a multiple case study in mathematics education. *Focus on Learning Problems in Mathematics,* 19(3), 1.

Reinhard, S.C., Horwitz, A.V. (1995) Caregiver burden: differentiating the content and consequences of family caregiving. *Journal of Marriage and Family,* 57, 741–750.

Room, R., Janca, A., Bennett, L., Schmidt, L., Sartorius, N. (1996) Cross-cultural applicability research on diagnosis and assessment of substance use disorders: an overview of methods and selected results. *Addiction,* 91, 199–220.

Roychaudhri, J., Mondal, D., Boral, N. et al. (1995) Family burden among long-term psychiatric patients. *Indian Journal of Psychiatry,* 37(2), 81–85.

Ruiz, N.T. (1995) The social construction of ability and disability: I. Profile types of Latino children identified as language learning disabled. *Journal of Learning Disability,* 28, 476–490.

Sartorius, N. (1976) Classfication: an international perspective. *Psychiatric Annals* 6, 22–35.

Sartorius N., Kaelber C.T., Cooper J.E., Roper M.T., Rae D.S., Bulbinat W., Üstün T.B., Regier, D.A. (1993) Progress toward achieving a common language in psychiatry: results from the field trial of the clinical guidelines accompanying the WHO classification of mental and behavoral disorders in ICD-10. *Archive of General Psychiatry* 50, 115–124.

Saxena, S., Dhawan, A. (1995) Editorial: Disability and burden of depressive disorders. *National Medical Journal of India,* 12(2), 49–50.

Schensul, J.J., Le Compte, M.D. (eds.) (1999) *The Ethnographer's Toolkit.* Walnut Creek, CA, Altamira Press.

Scheer, J, Groce, N. (1988) Impairment as a human construction: Cross-cultural and historical perspectives on variation. *Journal of Social Issues*, 44(1), 23–37.

Schmidt, L., Room, R. (1999) Cross-cultural applicability in international classifications and research on alcohol dependence, *Journal of Studies on Alcohol* 60, 448–462.

Sethi, B.B. (1980) Editorial: 1981–Year of the handicapped. *Indian Journal of Psychiatry*, 22(2), 127–128.

Shakespeare, T. (1993) Disabled people's self-organization: a new social movement? *Disability, Handicap and Society*, 8, 249–264.

Sheehan, D. V., Harnett- Sheehan, K., Raj, B. A. (1996) The measurement of disability. *International Clinical Psychopharmacology*, 11(suppl. 3): 89–95.

Shern, D. L., Trochim, W. M.K., La Comb, C.A. (1995) The use of concept mapping for assessing fidelity of model transfer: An example from psychiatric rehabilitation, *Evaluation and program planning* 18(2), 143.

Silveira, E., Ebrahim, S. (1995) Mental health and health status of elderly Bengalis and Somalis in London. *Age and Ageing*, 24, 474–480.

Spitzer, R. L., Kroenke, K., Linner, M. et al. (1995) Health-related quality of life in primary care patients with mental disorders: results from the PRIME-MD 1000 study. *Journal of the American Medical Association*, 274: 1511–1517.

Statistics Canada (1993) *Adults with Disabilities: Their Employment and Education Characteristics. 1991 Health and Activity Limitation Survey*. Ottawa: Ministry of Industry, Science and Technology.

Strauss, A.L and Corbin, Juliet M. (1994) *Basics of Qualitative Research : Techniques and Procedures for Developing Grounded Theory*, 2nd edition. New York, NY, Sage Publishers.

Thara, R., Raj Kumar, S. (1993) Nature and cause of disability in schizophrenia. *Indian Journal of Psychiatry*, 35(1), 33–35.

Thara, R., Raj Kumar, S., Valecha, V. (1988) Schedule for the Assessment of Psychiatric Disability: a modification of the DAS II. *Indian Journal of Psychiatry*, 30, 47–53.

Trawick, M. (1988) Spirits and voices in Tamil songs *American Ethnologist* 15, 193–215.

Trochim, W.M. K., Cook, J. A., Setze, R. J. et al. (1994) Using concept mapping to develop a conceptual framework of staff's views of a supported employment program for individuals with severe mental illness. *Journal of Consulting and Clinical Psychology*, 62(4), 766.

Trotter, R.T. II (1991) Ethnographic research methods for applied medical anthropology. In Hill, C.E. (ed.) *Training Manual in Applied Medical Anthropology*. American Anthropological Association Special Publications No. 27. Washington, D.C., American Anthropological Association.

Trotter, R.T. II (1995) Drug Use, AIDS, and Ethnography: Advanced Ethnographic Research Methods Exploring the HIV Epidemic. In Lambert, E.Y., Ashery, R. S., and Needle, R H. (eds.) *Qualitative Methods in Drug Abuse And HIV Research*. NIDA Research Monograph 157. USDHHS. Rockville, MD, National Institute on Drug Abuse, 38–65.

Trotter, R.T., Schensul, J.J. (1998) Methods in applied anthropology, in Bernard, H.R. (ed.) *Handbook of Methods in Cultural Anthropology*. Walnut Creek, CA: AltaMira Press. 691–735.

Tsuji, T., Sonoda, S., Domen, K. et al. (1995) ADL structure for stroke patients in Japan based on the functional independence measure. *American Journal of Physical Medicine and Rehabilitation*, 74, 432–438.

UNDP (1993) *Human Development Index*. Geneva: United Nations Development Programme.

Üstün, T.B., Chatterji, S. (1998) Editorial: measuring functioning and disability – a common framework. *International Journal of Methods in Psychiatric Research*, 7, 79–83.

van Meter, K.M. (1990) Methodological and design issues: techniques for assessing the representatives of snowball samples. NIDA Research Monograph 98, 31–43.

Verschueren, J. (1995) The pragmatic return to meaning: Notes on the dynamics of communication, degrees of salience, and communicative transparence *Journal of Linguistic Anthropology* 5(2), 127–156.

Weller, S.C., Pachter, L.M, Trotter, R.T. et al. (1991) Empacho in four Latino groups: a study of intra- and inter-cultural variation in beliefs. *Medical Anthropology*, 15(2), 109–136.

Weller S.C. and Romney A.K. (1988) Systematic data collection. Sage University Paper Series on Qualitative Research Method (Vol. 10). Beverly Hills, CA: Sage Publications.

Westbrook, M.T., Legge, V., Pennay, M. (1993) Attitudes towards disabilities in a multicultural society. *Social Science and Medicine*, 36, 615–623.

Wiener, R. L., Wiley, D., Huelsman, T. (1994) Needs assessment: combining qualitative interviews and concept mapping methodology. *Evaluation Review*, 18(2), 227.

Wig, N.N., Sulliman, A., Routledge, R. et al. (1980) Community reaction to mental disorders: a key informant study in three developing countries. *Acta Psychiatrica Scandinavica*, 61, 111–126.

World Bank (1996) *World Development Report 1996*, Washington, DC.

World Health Organization (1980) *International Classification of Impairments, Disabilities, and Handicaps: A manual of Classification Relating to the Consequences of Disease*. (Geneva, WHO) reprinted 1993 with foreword.

World Health Organization (1992) *The ICD-10: Classification of Mental and Behavioural Disorders: Clinical Descriptions and Diagnostic Guidelines*. Geneva, WHO.

World Health Organization (1993) Programme on Substance Abuse, Guidelines for Rapid Assessment Procedures, WHO/PSA/91.14. Geneva, WHO.

World Health Organization (1994) *Qualitative Research for Health Programmes*, WHO/MNH/PSF/94.3. Rev.1. Geneva, WHO.

WHOQOL Group (1995). The World Health Organization Quality of Life assessment (WHOQOL): position paper from the World Health Organization. *Social Science and Medicine*, 41, 1403–1409.

Yoder, P.S., Hornick, R.C. (1996) Symptoms and perceived severity of illness as predictive of treatment for diarrhea in six Asian and African sites. *Social Science and Medicine*, 43, 429–439.